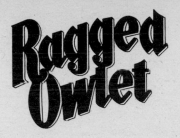

Ragged Owlet

*'YOU ARE DIFFERENT NOW AND ALWAYS
WILL BE DIFFERENT.'*
He said it gently, as to an equal, and his eyes
crinkled up in a sad smile. Nevertheless his
words had a suggestion of doom about them
which baffled me.

It was only gradually that I began to understand why I had been singled out: a label had
been pinned on me that April which I was to
carry for the rest of my life.

'Epileptic.'

Susan Cooke

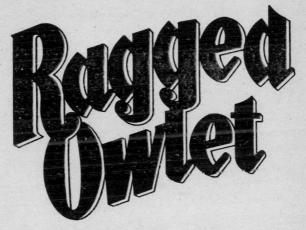

Ragged Owlet

The story of a young girl's
triumph over epilepsy

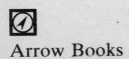

Arrow Books

Arrow Books Ltd
3 Fitzroy Square, London W 1 P 6 J D

An imprint of the Hutchinson Publishing Group

London Melbourne Sydney Auckland
Wellington Johannesburg and agencies
through the world

First published 1979
© Susan Cooke 1979

Set in 10/11 Press Roman by BSC Graphics, London

Made and printed in Great Britain by
The Anchor Press Ltd. Tiptree, Essex

ISBN 0 09 919040 0

Prologue

No one else could tell this story — not even another epileptic. We are all different. The origins of our single disorder differ widely. So does the extent of its effect upon us. But we all have the same problem of trying to hide it from everybody — friends, employers and government officials; or, having told the world, of taking the consequences, if we are strong enough. Because once you breathe the word *epileptic* you stand out like the Joker in a hand of gin rummy. Your hearers put you into a little box marked 'Beware', for the confines of general understanding about epilepsy are remarkably small — in some cases too small even to allow a struggle for acceptance, for equality in an emancipated Western society. That's what I found for many years. But it need not be like that. It's definitely worth the struggle. If you're game, there's only one thing that really matters — your own view of yourself, as a whole person.

This is not really a success story. But I reckon I've made a much more interesting mess of my life than many 'normal' people. The struggle continues for me and I only hope that my story will give others courage to fight their way out of a fenced-in, stigmatized position, and really *live*.

1

It was a bright day in late April, cool enough for us to be dressed in the regulation winter uniform of green tartan pinafores and gold blouses. Two prefects called me out of the classroom and told me that the Headmaster wished to see me. I knew why, more or less, but still felt a shiver of apprehension — all 600 of us stood in great awe of our Headmaster.

He was a small, strong man with a quietly compelling manner. Deeply religious. Highly thought of in the Protestant community and in charge of one of the most prominent private schools for girls in Melbourne, Australia. Under his direction, the enrolment had soared; so had the new blocks of classrooms. As well as being a Reverend he was also a Doctor, which I thought might be the reason he had sent for me now — genuine interest mixed with duty.

The new gravel scrunched under our feet as I walked under escort to the Head's study. Inside, I sat down, not even daring to look around at this sanctum which I had never entered before. He asked me what the doctors were doing for me. Told me I was still welcome at the school (that was puzzling) and, as far as he and the staff were concerned, their attitude towards me would not change (further bewilderment). He asked me what subjects I was doing in fifth form, what difficulties I might be having with them, what plans I had for the future. Having no idea where all this was leading, I murmured something about nursing and teaching. He seemed slightly impatient with my answers. That was not what he had meant at all. Well — whatever did he want me to say?

'You understand that your life will undergo a major change now. You cannot look on many matters as you used

7

to. You are different now, and always will be different.' He said it gently, as to an equal, and his eyes crinkled up in a sad smile. Nevertheless his words had a suggestion of doom about them which baffled me.

I said that I didn't see why anything should change. I would go on doing all the things I always did.

'You are a very courageous girl — very brave indeed,' he said with evident satisfaction.

But I wasn't really being brave at all. I was barely fifteen and, you see, no one had told me.

The Reverend Morley didn't feel it necessary to say the awful word. He must have presumed that I already knew and understood it and was probably suffering enough. Indeed, the class and the teachers had been primed not to mention this word to me, so I was unlikely to hear it at school.

Sick with horror, I heard him suggest that we should pray together for me in my new trial. One didn't say 'no' to the Reverend Morley. So, dazed and scared, I let him steer me, his hand on my shoulder, to the school chapel where we knelt down. Three or four times he urged me to pray out loud.

'Just a few words and Our Lord will understand.'

This was not something I could do in his august presence, even under normal circumstances. This time I honestly didn't know what I was supposed to pray for so I stared, with growing panic, at the supplicating figures in the stained-glass window. As we knelt there, the silence began to sing.

I sensed that Reverend Morley was displeased. For him, prayer would always be the ultimate solution to every problem. Frightened and uncomprehending, there was nothing I could do to ease the situation. Finally the Headmaster said a few words himself, rose quickly and dismissed me.

But my mystification was only increased by the interview and my apprehensions began during it. The Headmaster didn't do this sort of thing very often. Apparently I was a special case.

It was only very gradually, not until perhaps fifteen months

8

later, that I began to understand why I had been singled out: a label had been pinned on me that April which I was to carry for the rest of my life — 'Epileptic'.

An incident prior to this awful interview should have been a warning. But although the drama had taken place only two days before, it seemed fairly unconnected with the Headmaster's warnings. How could it warrant such red-carpet treatment?

The fifth form were in the school library for the afternoon, studying a little and passing notes to each other as conversation was forbidden. The next thing I knew, I was lying on the carpet in a dreamy haze, thinking that everyone else was doing the same. This strange, dream-like state must have gone on for some time. In moments of consciousness, when I tried to get up, I can remember the Reverend Morley's black cloak beside me and his hand holding me down. 'No don't get up, Susan', he said. 'Don't try to move,' Well then, I must just lie there. Not even the librarian, who was my sworn enemy, could overrule the Headmaster.

In between this unlikely dream that I was actually lying flat on my back during a school lesson, there were phases of complete oblivion. I had no idea what had actually occurred.

But Liz, my best friend, had been sitting at the table beside me . She had watched the whole thing. She saw me turn my head slowly to the right, then fall sideways, crashing into her lap. She thought I was trying to be funny until she saw my staring eyes and the stiffness of my limbs. Somehow she got me down on to the floor. My face turned blue; my body began thrashing and shuddering; my eyes began to roll and I was moaning horribly.

Liz was paralyzed with fear and convinced that I was dying. Being totally unprepared for what was happening, she felt her knees give way and she began to shake all over. She was appalled, revolted by this power that had suddenly possessed me, fought me and then departed, just as suddenly, leaving me apparently half-dead.

The poor librarian was undoubtedly just as frightened.

She sent for help immediately and, also fearing that I was dying, she sent to the top, which was just as well. Only the Reverend Morley could have been able to stop a roomful of adolescent girls going into hysterics of fear after witnessing one of their classmates undergoing such a violent and unaccountable illness. Liz has said that the unexpected shock left her shattered for over a week.

I remember very little about the rest of that day. A stretcher was brought and I was taken carefully down the wooden staircase and through the school grounds to the staff buildings. Two teachers took me home after my mother was rung. One of them advised her to get a doctor immediately as this had been more than just a fainting fit.

She must have been badly frightened and I often wonder how she felt that day. I was too dazed to notice her reaction, and just appreciated the warmth of my bed, the softness of the pillow for my throbbing head, and hot water bottle for my unusually freezing feet.

Nature is often kind to those she strikes down arbitrarily. To me she gave a complete state of blissful shock, lasting for several days after all of my worst fits. This enabled me to regain my composure without noticing what the rest of the world was thinking. By the time my mental energies were up to considering how other people were reacting to each fit, the effect had worn off on them.

And so I faced my wise and kind G P with no dismay, not even wondering why he had come. He prescribed emergency drugs immediately pending a specialist's report. He probably knew exactly what was the matter, as did the Headmaster, but although he had been our family doctor for many years, he explained nothing to my mother — possibly through fear of frightening her unduly.

For two days I lay in a state of unquestioning acceptance. When, on the second day, I was taken to a Collins Street specialist, I still didn't wonder why. I vaguely remember the brass name-plate reading 'Consultant Neurologist', which would probably have frightened me rigid if I had been up to considering its implications. There were the plush carpets, the silent lifts, the darkened waiting-room, the quiet-voiced secretary and the high-class magazines which mark the successful specialist's apartments. He was properous and greying with a bald dome. He sent me for several tests in order to confirm his suspicions.

One of the surest methods of diagnosing epilepsy is the use of the EEG (electro-encephalograph). It reads brainwaves and translates them on to a long sheet of paper which slowly unwinds while the pen-tracks go up and down. Neurologists can tell as much from that as heart specialists can from an electro-cardiogram (ECG).

The E E G is quite a formidable machine, and it was probably just as well that I was barely aware of what was going on during my first test on it. Nevertheless, it is not painful to have an E E G done. For a long time I believed that the flat electrodes which were attached to my head had needles in them — nobody enlightened me! First a hair-net was put on me, then the strategic points were rubbed with a fluid that conducts electricity well. Electrodes were placed all over my head, secured by a jungle of rubber tubing. Close your eyes . . . open your eyes . . . breathe deeply . . . close your right eye . . . now both eyes . . . hold your breath . . . It went on for an eternity (that is to say, about twenty minutes). Finally everything was undone and I could go — looking like a pale tree with a bird's nest on top. The first thing I did when arriving home was to wash the sticky mess out of my hair.

I still don't enjoy having E E Gs, although the methods have been modified. Now you can sit up comfortably instead of lying flat in a darkened room. Everything is so cheerful and streamlined, although this is offset a little by the fearful introduction of bright lights flickering at differing speeds, which apparently gives valuable extra information.

The pen-tracks on the E E G machine showed me up as a classic case with the typical epileptic patterns. I was not told this for some time, but I often glimpsed little bits of paper, extracts from the E E G, glued into my growing medical file and marked with lines in red ink. They must have spoken volumes to the neurologist.

From this point began the long experimentation to discover which combination of anti-convulsant drugs suited me best. They were all prescribed at various times — dislantin (epanoitin), ospolot, mysoline, tegretol and phenobarb. Little did I realize, when it all started, that, far from being discontinued after a few weeks as in all the other illnesses I had ever had, the taking of pills would go on for the rest of my life.

Once I had recovered from the fit and seen the specialist, there seemed no reason to stay away from school any longer. A growing awareness of other people's reactions after the first fit made it obvious that something about me had radically altered. But I couldn't fathom what it was. That's why the interview with the Headmaster puzzled me so much. I didn't think that I had changed overnight: those who did weren't going to tell me so in as many words.

But what had appeared to me at fifteen to be a bewildering and upsetting interview with the Head had in fact been a carefully planned part of the sequence of events following that first fit. Some of my teachers have expressed profound admiration for the way the Reverend Morley coped with the situation. I, as the patient, was having the easiest time just lying on the floor while the rest of the class believed I was really dying. Reverend Morley took complete control and, in his calm manner, was able to reassure the class immediately and later that day. Without this sort of positive leadership, coupled with a real background knowledge, many of the girls would certainly not have been able to come to terms with the phenomenon at all. Therefore, in retrospect, I have a lot to thank the Reverend Morley for.

To discover exactly what went on at school while I was passively allowing things to happen around me, I wrote recently to the Headmaster, who is now retired. In his reply, he described his reaction to that unusual and disturbing crisis in his school.

There was an urgent knock at my study door. This time it was a call to the fifth form group.

'It's Sue,' said the girl. Susan was subject to epileptic fits of the more serious kind.

Earlier on the situation had been talked over with the girls in Susan's class. She might suddenly need help. She could collapse at her desk and fall heavily. She could turn and thrash out with her arms, groan despairingly and clench her teeth. The two girls nearest to her should help her, the rest continuing with their studies. The helpers should gently but firmly restrain her and part her closed teeth with a pencil or ruler to prevent injury to tongue or lips. A third girl should go for help to the sick-room or to my study.

And that's how it generally happened. I would quickly be on the scene to find that the first steps had been taken. The study group would be tense but outwardly intent on reading. Then presently the quietness of the calm after the storm, and the awakening — the pale, intelligent face, so surprised, so wondering — so exhausted — with the words, 'What happened?' 'Where am I?' Then the stretcher to the sick-room and the phone call to home and the soft bell for the change of lessons.

I always marvelled at the simple pattern of behaviour of all concerned, especially the girls of the class. There was always someone doing the right thing — this sense of outgoing concern and hope. Not much discussion. Perhaps something like, "Not as bad as the last one."

And always that utter surprise on Susan's face as her eyes opened again and soon the words, "What happened?"

The girls were always asked to co-operate with the teachers in any new situation and were expected to act like adults when any crisis arose. I believe I was the only epileptic-type crisis to date, but other cases — such as girls who had lost a parent or were having adjustment difficulties — were discussed between the class and their teachers or the Headmaster, and then dismissed. For two years our class included a mentally handicapped girl. We were all told that she was coming to us — and even why she was coming. All exceptions were enfolded in the structure of the class, and each class looked after its own. Therefore, when my case came up before them, all thirty-six of those sixteen-year-old girls would have been at least responsive to such discussion and prepared to accept the possibility of further, similar incidents.

So, quite without my knowledge, there was a simple first-aid system always ready to go into operation while I was at school. Whoever was in charge of a class would silently indicate the two girls who were to be 'helpers' and it was understood that these girls were to look after me in the event of a fit. I don't know whether the helpers resented being chosen, because no word was ever breathed to me of this system and I was never aware of any action that must have occurred eight times a day. I give the school full credit for absorbing such a constant and disturbing crisis into the everyday life and understanding of hundreds of teenage girls. Reverend Morley was always there within minutes of an attack. I grew to recognize the presence of his black gown beside me, as a fairly sure indication that yet another fit had taken place. Perhaps he came principally to calm down the class but my trust in him grew as my awe lessened.

In this well-regulated atmosphere I had no reason to fear being singled out or avoided. For a long while I was not even conscious that there could possibly be grounds for such avoidance; I could not see how my fits looked to the other girls. Children are not as cruel as is commonly believed, especially if the reasons for consideration are explained to them.

I have never seen anybody in any sort of convulsion. Perhaps this is fortunate — perhaps not — but in a way I hope that I never do. In the early years, seeing someone in a fit might have given me a better standpoint from which to judge the probable extent of the impact on those around me. But it might also have given me a complex. It was harrowing enough watching my mother have a seizure due to a blood clot. I dreamed about it for years.

By all accounts the appearance of someone in a fit is quite terrifying until the onlookers get used to the idea. My mother, who saw me in so many fits, has never got over the shock of what I actually look like; perhaps she finds it worse because she feels more closely involved.

In a major epileptic fit (commonly called *grand mal*) what happens to me is this: my eyes go glassy and from then on I am unconscious. My head turns slowly to the right (the muscles in the left side of my neck usually complain for a day or two afterwards) and my body becomes rigid and falls sideways. All the muscles are taut, but I don't feel any pain. The fall usually means a big lump on my head, and bruises on my left arm, shoulders, ribs and hip, varying in degree depending on how far I have fallen. It is rather like a stroke, a kind of death-in-miniature. Because I am not breathing, my face turns blue and saliva trickles out of my mouth. If it happens during the night my pillow is always wet.

This lifeless condition may last for thirty seconds or a minute and, until the seizure breaks, to an onlooker it looks far more serious than it is. Then breathing begins again very heavily, causing the saliva to blow through clenched teeth and giving the typical appearance of foaming at the mouth. The rigidity gradually leaves my muscles, to be replaced by the 'thrashing and gnashing' stage. My teeth grind together with almighty strength. My tongue is usually badly bitten on the left side — the side to which I always fall. This gnashing is so strong that onlookers are advised to avoid the patient's mouth; my mother has had some badly bitten fingers in her attemps to save my tongue.

The alarming thrashing about of the body is normal in *grand mal*. But only we know why it happens. For me it is because I have been burried at the bottom of a black ocean or in a grave (the eyes, although wide open, can't see anything but blackness because the brain is not receiving visual messages during a fit) and I frantically try to reach the surface and light again. Every muscle in my body is used in this intense effort, this struggle for life.

Finally the brain begins to function more normally, but it is a slow process. In my case it takes two or three hours to discover where I am (at home, at school, which country, city, building) because everything around me is unrecognizable. I don't know the time, the day, whether it is morning or evening, where I should be (at work? in bed?), or what I was in the middle of doing. It also takes quite a while for me to realize that I've had a fit at all; other people's reactions or, as at school, the presence of the Reverend Morley during school fits, helps, but it all takes much longer when I am alone. The final results are a splitting headache, a swollen tongue, an inability to balance, extreme cold and a problem with focusing my eyes — plus an overwhelming desire to sleep. The intense physical effort needed to swim up from the bottom of my ocean (the animal instinct to survive, I suppose) has quite exhausted me, so — as on that first day — I lie passively while everything happens around me.

After several hours, I can again think more clearly and the headache may be reduced to a more tolerable feeling of fragility all over my body. My chest muscles often hurt as a result of their ordeal and it takes a long time to organize the most ordinary daily tasks. After a milder fit, I usually take up the daily programme, but a serious *grand mal* can completely write off one or even two days.

A seizure of this kind is a common enough experience for thousands of people all over the world every day. In Great Britain alone, there are 3000 new epileptics diagnosed every year; 400,000 altogether. Some of us have even become famous — Dostoevsky, Napoleon, Julius Caesar, not to mention that well-known cricketing personality, Tony Greig.

Thank God I remain continent; some epileptics become incontinent during their fits, which must add to their own and their onlooker's discomfort and embarrassment. My fits vary greatly in degree, but the above is a general description of a *grand mal* or major convulsion — the reason why serious epileptics have been locked away or shunned by 'normal' people since the beginning of time.

From the time of that first fit, I was taught to distinguish between a *grand mal* and what the specialist called *petit mal*. It is quite probable that I had been experiencing *petit mal* for several years, for at school I had been labelled as inattentive and a dreamer; fortunately I made up for this by success in examinations. I would often gaze out of the window and fix my attention on the blue sky, to the annoyance and exasperation of the French mistress or the arithmetic mistress, who may have just scolded me for the same thing five minutes earlier. It was a small compensation, I suppose, that I finally had an excuse for such rudeness.

Grand mal can be described as an electrical storm in the brain which causes a sort of short circuit, temporarily knocking the patient out like lightning. *Petit mal* is a gentler electrical storm which doesn't floor the patient but just causes the mind to seize up for several seconds. All memory of what one is supposed to be doing is wiped out and it may take five or ten minutes to recover the thread of the conversation. It is rather like plain absent-mindedness. I found that with a *grand mal* people could see that there was something definitely wrong, and they accepted that I might do anything as a result. But during *petit mal*, people are unaware of a physical cause and, with no knowledge of my medical history, they have every right to believe that I am being downright rude or lazy.

When I was first diagnosed as an epileptic, I was having about thirty minor seizures — *petit mals* — a day. I never actually counted them, but they could be annoying; usually they were brought on by somebody asking me a question at school, for example, but they happened just as often when my attention became riveted on something quite insignificant like a fence-post or a blade of grass. I had a sort of total concentration, an unbreakable absorption in tiny events.

Luckily for me, teachers and family were soon geared to

17

this happening, but many children experience these seizures, undiagnosed, for years and are upbraided for being inattentive, just as I was. Fortunately, again, my earlier education did not appear to suffer from the presence of *petit mal*. Many children write themselves off early as 'hopeless' or 'stupid' because they simply fail to hear or recognize a teacher's instruction or question; or worse, they might understand but be physically unable to answer the exasperated adult at the moment.

These were the two varieties of my new 'condition' which I was first taught to recognize and report to the neurologist. Yet the work 'epilepsy' had still not entered my vocabulary!

It became a common sight — me being carried through the school grounds on a stretcher, smiling weakly at anyone whose eyes I met in a moment of consciousness. But there were many fits in the evenings, also — especially in front of the television. And there were some in the mornings, under the shower.

We soon cottoned on to the fact that any play of light was likely to start me off — even the reflected sunlight on the windscreen of a passing car, seen through the venetian blinds. So the strong Australian sun, reflected off the wall and through the continually falling water near the shower head, was a frequent beginning to a proper *grand mal*. Well — I wasn't going to stop having showers. My mother got used to hauling me out, slippery and dripping, on to the bath mat. Here my guardian angel has been watching, because I've never had any serious accident in the shower or bath. Baths, in Australia, were more of a luxury, partly because of the necessity to save water. I gradually discovered that a long, hot bath could be just as dangerous as a shower in precipitating fits. I love them hot. But the heat and resulting steam (which probably prevents me from getting enough oxygen) often causes a succession of *petit mals* and I have had at least one *grand mal* while alone in the bath, only just escaping drowning.

Television was initially a frequent cause of *grand mal*. Strangely enough, we were not told this, but were left to find out by trial and — frequent — error. Australia only had black-and-white television for many years, and it's possible that the quality of the picture was not as clear as that in the United Kingdom or America. But studying for the Leaving Certificate (fifth form) was a serious business so I didn't watch much television. Besides that, Australian television standards were rather wanting. British films and comedies were a rare treat in the midst of all those American programmes that had been churned out in the fifties and sold to the A B C when America had finished with them. On the whole I preferred talking to our adorable black mongrel dog on the back steps.

I soon learned to avoid flickering lights, especially fluorescent ones. They seemed especially dangerous, with their 'whiter' light and accompanying buzz. Presumably the cinema was even worse, but we were not in the habit of going into the city to see a film more than once or twice a year. The local cinemas, where I had lined up with my threepence to see cowboy films as a child, had been closed several years earlier and given over to the more profitable business of squash or ten-pin bowling.

By the time the film '2001' came to be shown, I was well used to avoiding the sort of things which sparked off a fit. And when it came to the long section made up almost entirely of flashing lights, psychedelic colours and other hallucinatory effects, I literally ducked under the seat.

If I had envisaged how many adjustments in my life and that of the family would be needed, and just how much there was to learn about this new element in my life, I might not have appeared nearly so courageous in the eyes of the Headmaster.

2

The onset of epilepsy is so startling that at first it seems as if nothing will ever be the same again. Suddenly, I was jerked into a totally new way of life. Many radical changes became necessary.

An epileptic must learn to make each day into a regularized, almost regimented sequence. The most important factor is to take the right amount of drugs without fail. I was also advised to 'eat little and often' in order to maintain regular levels of blood-sugar. Almost as necessary is a minimum of eight hours sleep. The phenobarbitone which was immediately prescribed is apparently necessary to calm me down and prevent too much brain activity. It has never made me feel less energetic but it does ensure that I get enough sleep. Otherwise I go around all day like a bear with a sore head. There is little chance of me ever becoming an insomniac.

The eternal round of regular hours, sleep, food, drugs and the increasing watch on many new factors which might cause a *grand mal* could have been extremely irksome. But was life going to be indeed so very different? Even before I was diagnosed as an epileptic, I had been forced by circumstances into a quiet and somewhat solitary existence.

When I was six, my father left home and took my loved elder brother with him. But he had no intention of neglecting the two of us left with our mother. So, during the week we lived rather uneventful lives at home, whilst every second weekend was spent equally quietly on my father's small farm. As children we were left to follow our own childish occupations. We were all individuals with varying interests and didn't often play with each other, but at least we were together regularly. Peter helped my father on the farm and practised athletics, Michael went out shooting and became a philosopher, while I worked at the garden, read Dad's books and listened to all his old classical 78 rpm records, mainly Beethoven and Tchaikovsky, on a hand-wound gramophone. Much later, when electricity finally reached our area and we got a radiogram, I grew to love Chopin as well.

I was terribly moody and often at the mercy of extremes of happiness and sadness. There were times when I would stand on our large, airy verandah and become totally absorbed in the glare of the sun on the silver blue gums, shiny with eucalyptus oil. Sometimes I would find myself half a mile from the house with no memory of walking there and no reason to go, particularly as there was a great danger of snakes, even in the garden. Any of these small episodes could have been the beginning of *petit mal*.

Peter and I had horses which we rode on most afternoons in the surrounding countryside. We learned bush-lore at an early age and would often spend weekends exploring the virgin bush on our own or building bridges together across the gullies. Some of these were quite daring structures, twenty feet long and fifteen feet from the ground with three or four trestles. Peter designed them and cut the logs; I hung on to the ends of the block and tackle which raised the logs, and fetched squash and biscuits from the house. It was a useful partnership. We had no friends of our own age and we didn't miss them, but I found this a handicap later on, not having a clue where to start with a member of the opposite sex any more than with one of my own. While learning much about the natural world I was learning very little about human interaction and response.

Both my parents lived extremely quietly. There was almost no socializing. My mother was busy with small children and felt extremely alone in Melbourne after my father left, as all her family and friends were in Sydney. Surburban Melbourne is still not the friendliest of places for anyone without an established social life. My father had become deaf at an early age and, after some conflict, he must have found solitude the happiest state. His interests were equally divided between his small company of chartered accountants and the tranquillity of his beloved Australian bush.

Weekends at home were spent playing the piano, walking the dog, going to church, reading and other solitary occupations. School work, needlework and a discovery of classical music occupied my weeks so I was already leading an extremely quiet, well-regulated, unexciting life at fifteen. This proved to be an unexpected advantage. Whereas another teenager might have found that the imposition of a new set of rules cost them much wailing and frustration, it was virtually lost on me.

It still amazes me how I managed to go for so long without thinking of the implications of the whole business. Realization came very slowly and gradually, yet the adults (and probably most of my classmates) at school and at home must have looked on me with quite new eyes – with fear, compassion, uncertainty, suspicion or acceptance, depending on their tolerance, knowledge and experience. It certainly made a vivid impression upon them as they can all remember having seen me during fits. One of my favourite teachers admits to being terrified in case she couldn't perform the necessary actions. They had been told that separating my teeth was vital although it was later found that the best thing to do, apart from removing any objects which I might bang into during the thrashing stage, was simply to leave the fit to take its own inevitable course.

The same teacher, however, forgot to be frightened when I was actually present. It was encouraging to learn that she seldom even considered the likelihood of a fit occurring while she was in charge – until it did happen, and then my classmates were much more useful at acting nurses. Another teacher, having a good friend who was an epileptic and also coming from a medical family herself, was not unduly apprehensive and was able to dismiss her qualms more easily. The teachers were, after all, only human and must have experienced a whole range of natural reactions. It was their complete success in hiding it from me that I admire so much.

People at school soon got used to the phenomenon. Liz, who was closest to me, said that for a few months our relationship, at least from her side, did not have the same equilibrium. She was confused and scared, which hindered her feelings. So it took her a bit of time to get used to this totally unexpected event and what was to follow. Then she became what she describes as 'more rational', and she was able to accept the fits as a physical illness.

I expect that the basic diet of the New Testament did not help at first. Many of the girls knew the Bible stories off by heart, so it must have come as quite a shock to find one of those people possessed by devils, whom Christ exorcised, actually transported into their own classroom. It would have taken some effort for them to rationalize in the way Liz did, such violent and alien attacks as being entirely physical, and I suspect that some of the girls never could. But like most school classes they were a loyal group, unlikely to reject any member, however odd, except for a gross breach of their own particular code of honour. Liz went further than plain acceptance. After a bit of basic research she discovered in I can't think what book that highly sensitive, intelligent people were more susceptible to epilepsy, so she became defiantly proud of my friendship and defended me to the others while I was extremely grateful for hers.

The school was a good place for an unconventional child. The gentle, religious atmosphere fostered a spirit of charity in the girls and there was no question of jeering or ridicule. I was much younger than most of my classmates, having started primary school at the age of three instead of the customary five, which was still possible for an eager child then. Therefore my social development was not as advanced as that of classmates. Some had regular boyfriends, most went to frequent parties and many were depressingly pretty to my undiscriminating eyes. The fact that I usually beat them in exam results was small compensation for my woeful lack of hangers-on.

Being diagnosed as an epileptic was soon to become a sort of excuse for this growing social inferiority. It was not that I wanted to be different; quite the opposite — my inability to think and feel the same as these girls was a source of tremendous unhappiness. But Liz was not like them. She was from a sheltered, puritanical home in the middle of the wheat belt, in a small town on the Murray River. She also felt something of a misfit in this class of sophisticated city girls. So she was drawn to another misfit — me. I have her word for it that I was always 'different', even before becoming an epileptic, but she preferred me that way. This is an important point. Perhaps the onset of epilepsy did not change my personality as much as I came to believe. Perhaps it was, indeed, only an excuse that I pounced upon whenever necessary, to explain away the differences, real and imagined, between myself and the rest of the class.

The continuation of the fits neither gained nor lost me any friends. Very soon the teachers would accept no nonsense from me and the class became accustomed to the much-needed diversion twice a week or so. My only reaction initially was to drop geography — weather and rocks were boring and there were only five passes needed to proceed to the matriculation form. This was the first, but not the last, sign of my giving in to the epilepsy. If I was going to have frequent fits at school there might not be time to catch up on all the work which I missed. I could have coped easily with the course but my mother, not understanding the disorder and having at first only dim notions of my condition as being associated with mental illness, was frantic with concern. She felt the pressure of studying would make me worse. In fact, this was the only area of

24

life where I felt really confident.

There were other small changes. After the first couple of fits I was advised to wear an identification bracelet with name, telephone number and drugs inscribed on it. This is probably a good idea for epileptics who may have frequent day-fits in public and take a long time to come round, but I found its main effect was to single me out. We were strictly forbidden to wear jewellery at school, I received a special dispensation which I enjoyed — for a short time.

Another distinction which I enjoyed was going out in the middle of a lesson, precisely at noon, to take my pills. Apart from that (and dropping geography), I didn't use epilepsy as an excuse at school, because I liked lessons and didn't particularly want to avoid work. But I was withdrawn from the school play that year, in case I had a fit on stage. Fair enough. We were doing J.M. Barrie's *The Admirable Crichton* and I was to be the young minister who chased a maid called 'Tweeny' among the bamboo of a desert island. It was not a very big part but the dangers were too obvious — not so much to me as to the play. If one of the characters was suddenly stricken on stage, the whole audience might have to forgo the dubious pleasure of the rest of the performance.

It didn't occur to me that my social life might be jeopardized, that my career prospects might be radically altered or that my chances of 'marriage and a family' were low, this last being the ultimate aim of most Australian girls or, at least, so it seemed to me then. My knowledge of the implications for someone with epilepsy, especially in Melbourne with its left-over Victorianism and even remnants of superstition, was nil. Therefore the prayer of the Reverend Morley was lost on me, even when I did learn to call myself by my new name.

It was to be many months before my mother, my closest relative, would begin to learn the truth about my condition.

Much of her information was finally gathered from neighbours. It was possibly years before she was told its name, let alone what it might do to change me, so she was in no position to discuss these matters with me. Meanwhile she had to cope with the fits, often three times a week, and sometimes twice in a day, without having much idea as to the cause, the probable duration or the seriousness of these 'turns', as she was taught to call them. Nobody enlightened her, either.

Perhaps my mother's worries and fears could have been alleviated by a bit more communication with the doctors and teachers who were looking after me. Apparently she was never invited into the interviews I had with the doctors, so a few quick words were virtually all she had with them. It is possible that the school, the neurologist and the G P each assumed that someone else had explained the situation to her, but that's a poor excuse for such a paucity of liaison between them. It would be small wonder if a parent in such a situation were to imagine all sorts of dire possibilities. Hopefully, communications have improved since then.

For doctors and specialists I was just one of thousands of cases they saw every year, and so it was inevitable that I would be treated in a casual manner, and that my mother's questions and fears would be glossed over. What they ignored was the fact that for our family I was the first case of epilepsy we had ever encountered. It would have been a help if they had considered that, and it would have saved much frenzied search in right and wrong places for the answers to calm my family's worries. Also, if my mother had been told about the first-aid system that had been built around me at school, she might have felt happier during school hours. But, again, no discussion was forthcoming. Surely it would only have done good for everything to come out in the open? Better the devil you know than the devil you don't know! My mother was left to struggle on alone, and without direction.

My father says that after his initial reaction of horrified disbelief and hoping that it would just go away, his next reaction was to demand a cause. It seems that in all cases of less well-defined illnesses (especially mental illness, in which category many people would naturally put epilepsy), parents and close relatives tend to search feverishly for a cause for several reasons — to show the way for a possible cure, to put the elusive disease in a box so that it is easier to live with, to eradicate the collective guilt of heredity. My father searched carefully through his own family records and the nearest he could get was an unaccountable suicide by his great uncle. There must have been some hurried contact between my mother, who had all the worry, and my father (remarried by then), who seemed to feel more than usually concerned about my illness. When I was younger, he would bring me books and games if I was too ill to visit him.

It was soon apparent that the news had been relayed around my relatives. They must have felt very concerned and possibly even implicated because they got together and sent me to the Collins Street specialist. There was no National Health scheme at the time but there was plenty of private insurance available. They discussed the findings amongst themselves but nobody told my brothers — or me. I don't know whether they discussed causes with my mother, but her second thoughts (after 'Why did it have to happen to me?') flew to the little she knew of her own family medical history. She drew a blank, also.

The search for the meaning of this new thing, which had suddenly come amongst us and seemed set to stay, had, therefore, to proceed without the help of the doctors or teachers. My father, an extremely intelligent man in many fields, had no knowledge in this one so he speedily set about getting advice and information. Both my parents found an exasperating wall of reticence surrounding the subject.

The history was not much help, even though epilepsy is one of the few illnesses that has been documented from Egyptian times. Some of the pharaohs are said to have had it, and one reported treatment of it was trepanning — boring holes in the skull — as long as the holes didn't kill the patient first! The Greeks called epilepsy 'the sacred disease' because the inexplicable suddenness of the beginning and ending of a fit seemed to imply some sort of supernatural visitation. But the sufferers were not persecuted then, only set apart. The New Testament documents several people who were possessed by devils (often plural) whom Christ, or the disciples, exorcised. Exorcism is a common practice in all religious forms from the most primitive to the mystic, and is still practised today in the Christian church. Whether the subjects for this violent exercise were, in former centuries, always epileptics is doubtful. But many written accounts describe symptoms of fits similar to my own. The supposed devils enter and 'possess' a person's body for a few minutes, appear to fight them and finally leave them exhausted.

But this didn't help my parents, in this modern world, to understand what was the matter with me. Persistent inquiries in medical circles did finally come up with some fairly reassuring facts as to cause. So — what is epilepsy caused by?

To be on the safe side, neurologists admit that they don't know the definitive answer, but research has revealed much that was not known when I was fifteen. Epilepsy is a chronic symptom of an injury to the brain. That is, it is with us all the time even though we are not always in convulsions. It is usually revealed as an unchanging pattern on the E E G, and shows itself by a violent electrical storm in the brain which rapidly gathers momentum to burst into a *grand mal*, or to produce other less striking visible alterations in the patient. Recently it has been publicized that epilepsy is a chronic symptom of something physically wrong with the brain cells, not a disease in itself.

Therefore, epileptics who are otherwise normal can start shaking off all the fear and superstition which links epilepsy with mental illness. Some people who are mentally ill also have epilepsy, in addition to their other problems. It must make the mental illness so much harder to deal with, when something as physical as a fit accompanies more elusive, but no less real, symptoms such as acute depression or mental retardation. The tradition of believing fits to be a sign of mental illness is so strong that many of us, even faced with neurological facts, still feel the unfairness of stigma.

My father discovered that all genuine epileptic fits, whether major or minor, are definitely caused by damage to the brain cells, so the next step was to look for possible sources of such damage. There were several possible explanations which would at least exempt the family from blame. For example, as a small child I had had pneumonia three times, running temperatures over 104°F, which can do considerable damage to an infant brain; but at the time of my early illness, lengthy fevers were not considered as causes of brain damage.

Another likely cause would have been any fairly serious head injury. My father remembered that once when he had been taking us to Melbourne Zoo, there was a minor car accident during which I bumped my head rather badly on the windscreen and received concussion. There had certainly been an opportunity for lasting damage. Recalling those events of my childhood, my father felt more able to close the file on 'cause' satisfactorily to himself and open the file on 'effect' — how it would change my life.

My mother's greater involvement must have meant many more sleepless nights. But she knew of an even more likely source of brain damage. Many epileptics discover that they were 'instrument babies' (born with the aid of surgical forceps). This was my case also. Grasping a delicate, unborn head with the curve of solid steel can damage the brain if the instrument is not used carefully. Of course, the design of forceps and the training of midwives has improved tremendously in the last twenty-five years and this may help greatly to reduce the number of epileptics in the community — except that it is more than made up for by the increase in the number of serious car crashes, another source of brain damage. Such accidents, as well as surgical forceps, can cause a lesion, or scar, on an infant brain — the weakness where later electrical short-circuits will occur if other factors are also present.

And there are just so many other, peripheral causes which add to the burden of the existing lesion and finally may cause epilepsy. The more my parents asked and searched, the more numerous became the possibilities, until it may have seemed as if nobody has any right to escape fits of some sort. But the reasons why the majority of people did escape we did not discover until much later.

Some of us are born epileptic and begin convulsions in infancy. Sometimes infants with mental retardation also have epileptic fits. This must be especially difficult for families to accept because the baby has not yet become for them a person whom they can love anyway. Unfortunately, a common reaction amongst such parents, as with those of all handicapped children, is a feeling of guilt. Many people feel that it must be their fault, to some extent, that such a thing has happened to their child. A mother's worries are obvious — should she have taken those drugs to relieve depression or discomfort? Should she have rested more during pregnancy? Could a forceps delivery have been avoided by her own efforts? Fathers have the more nebulous worries that they have somehow not assisted their wives enough or given them all their support during pregnancy. There is a never-ending line of possible and impossible 'ifs' making many parents feel responsible for any permanent damage to their children. Although so common, this feeling is quite unnecessary. Worse, if it continues and the child becomes conscious of it, it can lead to a permanent wall of mutual misunderstanding between the worried parents, who are trying to be helpful, and the resentful child who is not sure where he stands in the family because he has always been treated 'differently'.

Then there are those who begin seizures in childhood. These children are often 'highly strung' and many have above average intelligence. By now, personality factors can affect an existing brain lesion. A fastidious child can become infuriated by something which, to the rest of the family, is quite tolerable. A naturally fearful child can become unreasonably terrified if a playful dog jumps at him. A child who appears slow to adults may be a deep thinker, becoming totally absorbed in apparently uninspiring things, taking quite ordinary situations to heart.

Hyper-sensitiveness is probably inherited; other factors added to this may allow a latent tendency for epilepsy, the lesion on the brain, to finally show itself in fits. A high I Q may be intolerable to a child. Rapid physical growth can burn up too much energy. A hidden grief may become too much of a burden — heightened sensitivity in a child results in enormous delights, but enormous and unbearable sadness as well.

If some or all of these factors come together in a child with an existing brain lesion, then what used to be uncontrollable sobs of rage, shame or grief, can become electrical storms and develop into epilepsy. In my case, there was the fact that I had grown incredibly fast around the age of twelve; from being almost the smallest in the class I became, in just three years, the second tallest. Also, admittedly, my school results were pleasing, but I Qs were not much in fashion at our school so we didn't know what mine was. These factors alone could not possibly account for the fits. I had never had temper tantrums or any sort of convulsions before my first fit, so my parents had to keep searching.

A peak time for the onset of convulsions is during the middle teen years. A new factor has come in here — the strain of adolescence. An American specialist has recently stressed that the young adolescent age group is especially vulnerable to epilepsy if the children are subjected to deep distress over a long period, and harassed by family upheavals. I was an extremely placid child. One grandmother often tells the story of how I would sit for hours on her lap when she took me visiting, never wriggling or interrupting, but watching all the goings-on with great seriousness. Perhaps I was too placid. My parents' separation when I was only six, their subsequent divorce and my elder brother going away to live with our father seemed to have no emotional effect on me. Perhaps one need look no further for a suppressed grief to add to other factors which finally burst into epilepsy when I was fifteeen.

There is no question that what happens to the body during adolescence affects most people's moods and personality. It may have been the last straw for me. I began having my periods at the age of twelve. When the fits settled into a pattern, I found there was always a bad one just before or during a period. There are extra drugs for these cases as well — it is quite a common experience amongst epileptics.

By the time the probable causes in my case were added up, my parents were able to accept it all with a bit more resignation and a bit less trepidation. In a way it was lucky for me that I became an epileptic when I did. Some people are finally diagnosed long after adolescence. What was the last straw in their case? Pressure of work or family? An imperceptible breaking-down of brain cells to uncover a lesion that had existed since birth, making it subject to electrical storms? A motor accident?

For these people it must be much more difficult to become reconciled to a new way of life than for those of us who get used to forgetting about it when we are much younger. Older people might have good careers which are jeopardized by the new revelation. They might fear the reaction of family and marriage partners, not to mention friends. For most it is a well-guarded secret; the stigma attached to epilepsy is much greater than with any other disease except mental illness.

I know at least one lady who is a noble exception to this business of secrecy and stigma. At fifty-eight she was finally diagnosed as an epileptic and the relief was amazing. That explained everything . . . and it did. For as long as her family could remember, she was liable to strange lapses during which she might pour tea deliberately and carefully over her daughter's head, or put the Sunday joint methodically in the rubbish bin, just as it was ready to carve. Her family had learned to put up with these 'queer turns'. But an extra amount of family stress finally exploded into a series of *grand mals*. So she was, of course, eventually diagnosed as an epileptic with the typical E E G pattern. At last she could see a valid medical reason for her continuing peculiarities; the transformation of her self-image is heartening!

Eventually, my family discovered another piece of information: there is no cure for epilepsy. But many people simply grow out of their fits and a combination of drugs can prevent all but the most serious fits. My parents kept on hoping that I would be one of the lucky ones. As for the real causes, many of these are still only speculation. What was, in history, called the Sacred Disease remains an enigma.

3

It is quite possible, even in this age of good drug-control, for parents and friends to be ruled by various fears and doubts, mainly due to a deplorable lack of general knowledge about epilepsy. There are some extreme cases, one of which was a major factor in the writing of this book. It is the story of a woman in Wales.

Like some other families, hers is still so ashamed of having an epileptic in their midst that they hide the fact with great determination. Since the age of thirteen this girl has never left the house, not even to go to chapel. She is the same age as I and has *grand mal* only slighly more often than I do. She is a prisoner, still, of her family's understandable fears for her, but less excusable shame for themselves. Some people tend to believe that their epileptic children will gradually deteriorate until they have to be transferred to an institution where they will eventually die. What a sad piece of judgement! It would surely surprise nobody if this poor woman whose home is her prison did become deranged.

Whether such fears entered the heads of either of my parents is hard to tell now. I would have expected them, never having encountered such a case before, and receiving little information from the doctors, to have at least thought of such a possibility. It was natural for them to want to protect me and treat me carefully, at least until they knew how serious the epilepsy might become. My mother had no way of knowing what the outcome would be, so perhaps extreme caution was in order. But she hadn't realized the miracle that modern medicine can perform with this and many other previously dreaded diseases. Also, she hadn't bargained with me.

Like many teenagers, I did the opposite to my mother's wishes as a matter of course. I had been labelled 'defiant' for as long as I could remember. Her suggestions, though often quite sound, all fell into one category for me — the wrong one. Anything from 'Get your hair cut' to 'Please don't ride your horse any more — what if you had a fit in the saddle?' was strategically ignored for as long as possible.

In the beginning I certainly needed the comfort and reassurance of my own bed and so I submitted to her ministrations gratefully. Every time I had a fit at school she came to take me home. I would stagger on her arm across the playground to the car. My sense of balance is always haywire after a fit and I am likely to do myself more harm falling down stairs than I have done during the seizure. My head always ached furiously and I desperately would want to be sick. The felling of fragility and 'not-quite-with-it-ness' would remain for the rest of the day — all of which I accepted, for about three months.

Then I began to rebel and decided that all the fuss was unnecessary — it interfered with the task of living too much and I was beginning to find the dependence very irksome. So, later in the year I would lie in the sickroom for several hours and accept a cup of tea from a teacher. That helped to stop the nausea somehow. Someone was usually sent to keep me company — possibly to make sure that I didn't go into another fit. Liz would creep into the sickroom instead of going to the library and say 'How ya getting on, Susie?' I could at least grin when she was caught. Then, with her help, I would often stagger back to the classroom and would find myself able to take part in the lesson much better than anyone would orginally have thought.

Some measure of will-power was needed to overcome the desire to remain comfortably under the grey army blankets. The sickroom was a severe, uninspiring place, not a refuge for loafers. So, once the headache had lost its force and my sense of time and place were restored, I would ask to return. It would have been so easy to relapse into being a long-term semi-invalid, letting everyone do everything for me, having my Grand Excuse as a reason for inactivity. But the natural rebelliousness of any fifteen-year-old against a situation forced upon her from outside was stronger. So my own personal little devil and I reached a compromise — he could stay and possess me; I was going to ignore him.

But there was soon rebellion in a much more important field. Suddenly, many of the adventures and activities I loved had become dangerous. The trouble is, caution can be extended to include every waking minute! If an epileptic is likely to have a fit at any time of the day, it is terribly dangerous even to sit on a piano stool in case he falls over backwards and breaks his neck; not to mention riding a bicycle or a horse, or walking along the edge of a cliff, or swimming.

Well — that is one way of looking at it, I suppose. Such a careful person would end up sitting in an armchair, twiddling his thumbs just waiting to have a fit, meanwhile dying of boredom, self-pity and frustration. The business of danger can be viewed from another angle — you pay your money and take your chances. Very soon I was on the side of the desperadoes, becoming a genuine dare-devil. Of course it is a gamble and of course I've had some accidents, but not enough to warrant wrapping myself in cotton-wool. I began to take a sort of ghoulish pleasure in imagining what *might* happen if I did something. For instance, I could have an epileptic fit while riding my horse, fall off, catch my foot in the stirrup and be dragged to a bloody death. But that didn't stop me riding. We would go for long day-rides, exploring the surrounding Gippsland Hills together, along the white dust of the backroads. My enjoyment was never clouded because I never really imagined that I would have a fit while I was on her back; only, perhaps, when she was rolling in the shallow sandy creeks while I lay on the bank, watching her and eating the lunch I had bought in the saddlebags.

Climbing trees, cliffs, rocks and gullies was also a source of great pleasure. That could lead to another gory death but I am always consoled by the fact that I won't feel anything if I die during a fit, so I still climb trees and cliffs with undiminished delight.

My poor mother — watching, worrying, waiting for the worst — she must have suffered agonies while I was glorying in the joyful energy of the Australian surf. But I would have missed so much by giving in. The hazards are obvious — a fit in the middle of those beautiful, crashing waves could mean certain drowning. Crossing roads, climbing stairs — even cooking and working with tools could be crossed off the list of permissible occupations.

Was all this rebellion against so many precautions just bravado? A recklessness that showed my disregard for life and other people's feelings? Perhaps, on the other hand, it was an absolute necessity to prove to myself that all was still well.

Strangely, I never considered that any of this daring was truly dangerous. And the family were a help. I cannot remember being forcibly restrained from doing any of these things, only advised not to and watched with great anxiety. As a result I began to temper my imagination a little, becoming accustomed to being surrounded by a certain sort of danger. It was all to become a grand, psychological exercise in personal freedom — the sort of freedom that 'normal' people take for granted.

I was so well shielded from the long-term implications of my epilepsy that I never really troubled myself with the family's reactions — any more than I wondered what they would think when I used to have asthma so often. But being rather sensitive to slight alterations in social interaction, I was soon aware that the family, as a whole, was regarding me in a new way. My relatives are numerous and scattered. As with most Australian families they believed that I was their responsibility and they accepted me as such. But in some respects they overcompensated, making allowances and, sometimes letting me get away with murder. But then, sometimes, they might come right back at me, possibly to ensure that I didn't think I could always get away with everything.

There didn't seem to be a change in my brothers' views of me. I have dim visions of the younger one calmly eating an apple in front of the television without even a glance at his floored elder sister. A careful discussion with this brother has revealed quite a different aspect — the one I never saw. He was only eleven when I became an epileptic and he admits that the accuracy of his memories is hard to gauge. The most marked memory is the feeling of utter helplessness and emptiness when I 'took turns'. He was by no means unaffected or detached; this would have been the first observation of his life that the family experience was something more than the eternal happy-endings as depicted in half-hour television production. He says that the best he could do was to run feverishly around the house searching for some object to force between my teeth — something that would not shatter (or ruin my teeth!).

I don't know why everyone was told that my tongue was the most important thing. By the time the fit had taken over, that is within a few seconds, it was already too late. There is no persuasion will make an epileptic obligingly open his mouth while you pop a knotted handkerchief inside. Everything happens far too quickly — and we are just as likely to choke on the handkerchief as on our tongue. Tongues and the sides of the mouth, although they can be very sore for up to a week after a fit, are very good at regenerating themselves. The other piece of first aid which people seem to think necessary — that of attempting to restrain the patient during the thrashing stages — is even more misguided. I hate being held down — in my fuzzy state it makes me fight all the harder because I can feel the weight of the ocean pressing down on me, a terrifying sensation.

It was impossible for my little brother, who saw the fits so often, to feel unmoved at the spectacle. He doesn't remember feeling ashamed so much as demoralized or empty — helpless, I suppose. He came to look on these episodes as a temporary experience during which he and my mother performed the necessary tasks until I was back with them again. It was probably afterwards that he would sit down, exhausted, eat an apple and watch television again, at which point I would come to!

Michael was never told what was wrong with me except in the simplest terms, and indeed he says that he still doesn't really understand. But what he does certainly remember is that the family all believed that I would not have a 'normal' life, and that the most traumatic part would be my relationships with the opposite sex. This would account for the new looks they all gave me. The family, therefore, must have agreed with the Headmaster. What they mourned for me after their consultation with the Collins Street specialist, was my lost opportunity to find happiness Australian-style — a solid husband, three lovely kids, a 'triple-cream-brick-front-vanilla' (every Australian's dream-house) with clean carpets, all mod cons and a beaut car in which to litter the Dandenong Ranges every Sunday afternoon. If the onset of epilepsy has indeed helped me to avoid such a fate then it's possibly a genuine 'blessing in disguise'.

When I was fifteen, Michael and I were still visiting my father every alternate weekend. There was no television there, and not enough water for showers. Also, I was able to relax completely in the bush. So my father only remembers seeing me in a fit on one occasion. This was on the beach, when a passerby called his attention to me thrashing about on the sand and frothing at the mouth. Obviously the sun glinting on the sea had done its work. My father was unlikely to have seen the fit without the help of the stranger because his favourite occupation on the beach was snoozing, with his hat over his face.

Generally, my father had no opportunity to watch the

progress of the epilepsy and could only follow with great interest the doctor's search for the best combination of drugs. His visions for my future had to alter somewhat, and although he says now that there is no reason why I shouldn't marry and have children, I know that at the time he felt the same as the rest of the family — that I could no longer have a normal life.

But it was my mother who, seeing me in so many fits, was bound to react most strongly. If my father first felt shocked disbelief, she must have been quite stunned. Not only did she feel the enormous responsiblity of finding the best way to treat me. It was also Mum who nearly sacrificed all her fingers trying to save my tongue; Mum who picked me up from school with a sinking feeling of 'not again' after each fit; Mum who traipsed around all the specialists with me; and Mum who received all my ungracious, rebellious ingratitude. I sometimes wonder where she found the strength to cope with me at all. But she did.

She became naturally over-protective, tried to find out what she could about all sorts of fits from good and bad sources, was bombarded with gossip about what could be harmful to me, and got herself generally worked up about the whole thing. She had a good friend, a Christian Scientist, who wanted me to go to their meetings. Modern faith-healers have apparently cured epilepsy (as well as cancer), simply by the laying-on of hands and the absolute faith of the patient. If I had been supersitious enough, or perhaps devout enough, I might indeed have tried that way. But in spite of my strong religious beliefs during adolescence, I never could bring myself to believe in faith-healing through a medium — at least not for my own problem, simply because the presence in the brain of a physical origin for epilepsy is medically demonstrable. Faith may move mountains but the removal of the cause of fits by prayer smacked too much of the old spirit-devil idea for me.

How would most mothers act in such a situation? Mine

was saddened and sometimes even in despair. She felt that the burden of my possible ensuing insanity (only one of the points which the doctors didn't help her on) would be too great for her — but I only found that out much later. Constantly up against defiance and rebellion, she soon resigned herself to watching what became known as 'my health' (she could rarely bring herself to speak nearer the subject), and generally making sure she was around when needed. Sometimes I could see through to her fear; sometimes, in desperation, she would try to stop me from going on some dangerous escapade, by telling me how horrible I looked while in a fit. But in general, for a woman coming to face the fact of an epileptic child alone, and with no knowledge of the thing whatsoever, she didn't do so badly with me.

It must have been a hard decision for her to continue allowing me to go to school by train, for instance. Australian suburban trains travel for most of the year with their doors open, to cool the packed, home-going passengers. I will never know just how much worry she had in those first years; she didn't convey her fears to me at the time.

My father's relatives treated me gingerly at first. The loved grandmother who had held me on her knee when I was a too-saintly child didn't even try to understand and so ignored my new state, thank goodness. The Sydney relatives, my mother's family, took a conservative view and were extremely sorry about this new burden with which we had been landed suddenly.

The first Christmas we spent with my dear old Sydney grandmother, a fine and good woman, who drank at least sixteen cups of tea a day and was an excellent plain cook in the old style. There were always Christmas puddings in white, calico bags hanging from the rafters in her kitchen. She had been born on the goldfields in Western Australia, last century, and married to a young Yorkshire immigrant who went away to the First World War. She could also be described as a bit Victorian and with her I had the ill-luck to have two fits in succession one night, while watching television. Everybody was quite appalled; Grandma nearly had a heart attack and my mother was terribly upset. I was used to fits by that time and certainly didn't see the reason for all this fuss, but it did bring home to me the sense that I ought to be ashamed and afraid to be seen in a fit because it upset those around me. Therefore it was my mother's intention to shield me from the rest of the world and, more important, to shield the rest of the world from me. In the beginning she really believed that such steps should be taken. I don't think she believes that any more.

4

In those first years, especially, I sheltered behind the epilepsy — when it suited me. There was a constant conflict between racing beyond all reasonable physical bounds to prove myself as capable, more capable than the rest of the class; and using epilepsy to excuse myself in those areas of life where I considered myself a failure. The excuse was unnecessary at school. Having sailed through fifth form, the Victorian Leaving Certificate, I took up five subjects in sixth form to sit for matriculation (and university entrance) without any clear idea of what I really wanted to do.

Necessary absences from school diminished in number as a pattern of evening fits emerged. In fact I was so much improved and adjusted to the new drugs that a year after my first fit I tried for the school play again and became Mr Bennett in a stage rendering of *Pride and Prejudice*. Mr Bennett was a man of few words (that is to say, few lines) who sat on the stage and looked on sardonically while the women in the family went into and out of hysterics on the subject of marriage. My favourite line, as I sat in my father's coat and trousers was, 'Well, Lizzie. Here's a thing! Your mother will never speak to you again if you do not marry Mr. Collins — and I will never speak to you again if you do!'

For those of the family who came to watch the performance it was apparently quite traumatic. They knew that a fit could come at any time, and I give them and the school full marks for not conveying any of their fears to me. Michael vividly remembers watching the play, trying to follow the story line, but chiefly being anxious lest I should forget my lines during a *petit mal* or even have a proper *grand mal* on stage. He was profoundly grateful every time I made an exit and even more than usually pleased when the play was over.

The consideration of a career was postponed over and over again. Perhaps nobody wanted to discuss it. At school we all filled in university application forms automatically. But universities are not free in Australia and students have to put themselves through, depending on parents and holiday or part-time work, unless they are lucky enough to win one of the coveted Commonwealth Scholarships, which provide fees and a living allowance. One disappointment that brought me a second interview with the Headmaster and gave me a glimpse of future limitations, was being chosen for the school debating team — only to discover at the last minute that the inter-school debate would be televised live. The Reverend Morley had received instructions to exclude anyone liable to take a fit before the cameras. The glaring and shifting lights would have been quite a hazard, so I conceded them that point.

Gradually it dawned on me that I could never become an actress or have anything to do with television and probably even radio. I love theatre; a professional once told me that I was a born comic, which made me very resentful as I had no chance of pursuing any such career. Actually, it is most unlikely that I am a born comic at all. What that actress saw was far more likely to be a pro-duct of rebellious nonchalance. Michael, along with many others who knew me in those first difficult years, presumed that the uncertainty of epilepsy would greatly affect the spontaneity of my life. It did — but in an unforeseen way. Just as my father had done when he became deaf years before, I over-compensated and became impulsive to the point of recklessness. If acting was out for me, what else might not go the same way?

There were growing social problems. Just turned sixteen and convinced that I was plain and uninteresting (for a start I was far too tall and had enormous feet), I was increasingly aware of the boyfriend drought. Nobody had told me that a girl is just as attractive as she feels; all manner of beauty treatments won't improve her own personal attraction. So when I compared my social life with that of the other girls at school and found mine wanting, I hid obstinately behind the conviction that it was no use me falling in love because my prospects for marriage-and-a family (still virtually the only option open to Australian women) were bleak. Nobody had said so in as many words, not to me that is, and I was still unaware of my label. But there were sufficient grounds for me to believe that something was patently, permanently and incurably wrong with me.

Liz had gone to college and it was uphill work finding a substitute for her friendship. My increasing wildness, the result of many desperate attempts at over-compensation, tended to alienate me from the other sixth-formers who disapproved of all this wanton enthusiasm. I found that my sedate classmates, many turned eighteen, would not tolerate my reckless presence in their serious discussions. So I was generally lonely, ate lunch in the splended isolation of a playground bench and wandered around aimlessly during breaks, trying to look as if I was doing something important.

During lessons, my friend Meredith and I would participate wholeheartedly, to the amusement of our classmates, who were too genteel to raise their hands (or perhaps had neither questions nor answers). For a time the teachers admired my zest but ultimately it exasperated them — 'For goodness sake put your hand down and give someone else a chance!'

Finally came the school dance and that was a disaster. I swapped brothers with another shy girl and was thoroughly miserable. Life in general had not prepared me for the sight of all those self-conscious boys trying to look as if they were having a good time with their equally self-conscious partners, who were really giving each other points on their dress, hairstyle and the handsomeness of the guy on their arm. The best part was supper — lemon meringue pie.

Towards the end of this final year I must have become conscious of my label. That goaded me into trying to find out a bit more about it. Before the exams I had a long discussion with my Form Mistress on the subject of careers and just how much she thought would be closed to me. The result was a tentative application for nursing school, the same one as my elder half-sister had entered some years before. After all, I never really envisaged that I would win a place at the university. But nursing! Obviously, we were all uninformed as to the far-reaching effects of being an epileptic.

It was from this time that I really started colliding with the world. Being all set for rebellion, and feeling generally unsettled with the sudden addition to my identity, didn't make my adolescence any easier. It was certainly not helped by the side-effects of some of the drugs with which the neurologist was experimenting, either. Phenobarb, although universally used for the treatment of epilepsy, can cause irritation in some adolescents. I was apparently one of those unlucky ones which it affected and I would become incensed with rage at any small thing that might irritate me. Mainly the family suffered from this. But I was also suffering. My little devil had pulled down the fragile self-image I had found in my first fifteen years, shattered it and now stood with hands on hips, daring me to build it again if I could. The new factor of epilepsy just didn't help in growing up.

In short — I never went out, nor was I ever invited to parties. I attended church socials feeling (and therefore looking) totally inadequate. But could adolescence have been any different? Do epilepsy and the eternal taking of

46

drugs change one's personality? At the time I could think of only one excuse for my lack of social success! I was an epileptic.

All through the heat of early summer we studied for our final examinations. The smell of the flowers, on our lemon tree is now inextricably mixed in my mind with Shakespeare's *Hamlet* and the sight of a baby pumpkin will always remind me of the history of the convicts. The examination results were marvellous. I was one of only two girls in the school to win a Commonwealth Scholarship. But I was too young to be allowed university entrance — you had to be seventeen. So I had to begin thinking of an alternative. There was no getting around it — my school days were over.

The results also won me a place in the nursing school (they had not yet asked for a health record) but, again, I was too young to start nursing, so I was given a job in the hospital in the X-ray department. I wore a white gown with a red waistband and wrote people's names on their X-rays as these fascinating pictures spewed out of the big developing machine. So there I was, immediate work-needs fulfilled, launched doubtfully into the world.

My mother was absolutely dedicated to doing something for me. Her continued dedication in the face of my rebellion was astounding. She tried hard to get me to visit the Epilepsy Foundation in Melbourne, thinking that perhaps they might have some constructive advice about survival in an adult world. Finally I agreed to an interview. That interview was quite a shock.

The patient woman who courageously organized the whole foundation was herself a permanent cripple, confined to a wheelchair, and not a day over thirty. She was accustomed to dealing with the most difficult epileptic cases — people who have daily, uncertain and dangerous fits — and she would pull out all the stops to find them a job with an understanding employer. A small number of companies gave her freedom to try them for a vacancy; no doubt she had worked on them for years to get them to that stage. Otherwise, the most serious adult epileptics were given a place in one of the foundation's hostels with a workshop attached. There, at least, young people could be safe and at the same time meet lots of other people with similar problems. This would bring in a new common denominator not available in ordinary life. It might also tend to arrest self-pity and self-preoccupation, while fostering new interests and hobbies and a social life. Compared to this woman's usual interviewees I was extremely well-off. I knew it. There was nothing she could do for me. Someone with fairly good drug-control, especially with university entrance, was expected to have comparitively few problems.

So my grand blanket excuse didn't really hold water. I wasn't bad enough for a sheltered workshop. But I soon discovered that I was not welcome at the nursing school either. I steeled myself to think carefully about the future. Should I take up the unexpected opportunity of university?

They began all the arguments against such a venture. For a start, I was a girl. Australia is a man's society and ten years ago girls didn't go to university without a struggle unless their parents were academics. It was a waste of the country's money. Girls only went and got married, wasting their expensive education. Nobody in our family had ever been to university. They left school and trained for a profession or went into existing family businesses. There was no precedent for me to go. My father had six children in all; I was the fifth — and moreover, a girl.

Both of my parents were doubtful of the value of a university education for me. What was the use? It was only postponing the ultimate decision. My father drove me all over Melbourne one night trying to convince me of this. In fact, this was the only occasion when my father's bitterness at having an epileptic child was ever apparent to me. He was especially careful not to show those feelings, having had to struggle himself with the consequences of a disability since the age of nine, when he became deaf. His struggles led him to become 'dux' of Melbourne Grammar School as well as captain of football and cricket!

Thank goodness for my rebellious nature and for an eccentric aunt who suddenly became interested in me, encouraging me with much brighter prospects than I was beginning to think possible. To all the normal arguments like 'I can't do this' and 'I definitely can't do that' she would say 'Why not?' in the most challenging and final terms. Why not indeed? My vision widened, my self-esteem grew. I began to think.

Everyone was concerned for me, but our family code was independence so I couldn't count on financial aid. However, this obstinately professional-minded, independence-oriented family were, all unknown to themselves, a tremendous help. It was just because I was a special case that they were stumped for an answer to my career problem. They gave me up as a rebellious dead-loss and left me to it. So I was free! Free to be anything I chose. Or was I. But the grass was not so green, for epileptics of any propensity are barred at every level from a huge number of professions. Sheltered workshops and special homes for adult epileptics are excellent and necessary for those who have three or four fits a day and who really can't be left alone for fear of physical hurt. But that isn't most of us — or me.

If you exclude all aspects of the medical profession, public service, transport or driving, teaching, most work in factories with machinery, all responsible jobs dealing with the public or the care of children, managerial positions and even receptionist work, that just about leaves absent-minded professor or chambermaid (ground floor only for fear of falling out of windows on the company time). Unless we decide not to tell the employer. Many people get away with that, especially if they only have fits in their sleep, or had epilepsy as children and are now completely controlled by drugs. But at sixteen, the likelihood of me getting away with it was small, although increasing. On the other hand, to tell a prospective employer was a bad mistake. In Melbourne, ten years ago, employers would as soon take on an ex-convict, the stigma was so great. As far as they were concerned, 'epileptic' was on a par with 'loony'. I just hope they have improved a little, but a conservative, serious-minded society doesn't change that easily.

So there I was, almost totally free of family pressure as to a career and unafraid of their displeasure. Admittedly, it was a limited freedom because my imagination did not go beyond the accepted professions. But it was face-about with employers. Even with a degree the chance of a job would be virtuallly nil.

Try to put yourself in our place. Where do we go from there? What's the use of training for anything if employers will prefer *anybody* before us? How can we keep up morale and self-respect if we're the only ones who believe we are good for anything?

Without university entrance I might have trained for accountancy, insurance or the stock exchange if I'd enjoyed figures. But I didn't. My mother was a first-class shorthand typist and doubtless I might have been the same — but there rebellion set in again. It is obviously easier for us if we aspire naturally to a job which is 'safe', in a protective environment, where we are surrounded by plenty of enlightened people to pick us up. But where do you find such a job in Melbourne?

In fact I know of one epileptic who is a successful receptionist-telephonist; another, who hasn't had a fit for years, is a highly respected man with a key office job; and a third who is a successful practising solicitor. But a fourth who had an extremely responsible position until her disability was disclosed, was pensioned off at twenty-nine. Thus are we singled-out, branded — nearly always without real cause to my way of thinking. Surely employers realize that a person who is desperate to prove himself capable in a job will work twice as hard?

It was turning out to be more of a predicament than I

had envisaged. Slung between my own little devil and permanent unemployment, I gave up consulting careers officers, personnel managers, labour exchanges and all well-meaning friends and acquaintances. I chose to become the absent-minded professor.

5

But until I grew old enough to begin the long haul towards this pie-in-the-sky professorship, I had to be content with manual work in the Royal Melbourne Hospital. There were certainly some advantages in this. For instance, I could finish with the Collins Street specialist at sixteen guineas a visit and go to the hospital neurologist any time I wished — for free.

Dr Ebeling was young, brilliant and impatient. He was tall with red-curly hair and did not have a bedside manner. We did not get on at all but it is possible that he did the most good for me that way. He would not allow self-pity. How many fits since the last appointment? Spots before the eyes? Dizziness? Anything else to report that was relevant? How were the new drugs affecting me? I gave up taking a written list of complaints to him. No simple, vague complaints were tolerated — Dr Ebeling was not paid to listen to stories of headache, fatigue and sore toes, but only facts bearing directly on the case.

This refreshing new doctor took a keen interest in me, as in all his patients. As a result I began to take more interest in myself and started to ask questions. So far I had never tried to find out what was really the matter with me, nor looked for any books on the subject. I had just allowed the doctors to do what they wanted, accepting everything that happened to me. But now came a surge of curiosity; I demanded to know what it was all about. And, simply by asking, I discovered quite a lot.

At first he asked me many questions which I had not been asked before. Did I experience an aura? An aura is a foreknowledge of the gathering storm which many epileptics have, sometimes in time to act upon it, stop what they are doing and lie down.) No — I had never experienced any such aura. My fits are over before I have the slightest knowledge of their coming, which makes life a bit more dangerous, as will be seen. On the other hand, it prevents me from going around and imagining auras, which could lead to a much greater preoccupation with self.

Did I experience focal attacks? I didn't realize there was so much variety to epilepsy. I had to ask him what that was, too. Focal epilepsy, apparently, shows itself as a tic or twitch. I was rather glad to discover it has a name because I used to get focal epilepsy often. It affected my right eyelid and can still be embarrassing. When I am talking to people it doesn't really help if that eyelid starts jerking away of its own accord. But this type of minor seizure can at least be disguised. It is a simple matter to rub the annoying eyelid and pretend that I am thinking deeply, or smile and wink daringly at the same time. It soon goes away.

I told Dr Ebeling about the frequency of *petit mals*. Could anything be done to reduce them? So many small seizures each day could be more than a nuisance if I was to go to university. *Petit mal*, I discovered, was the name given to minor childhood seizures. The doctor recommended more experimentation with drugs — a slow process, because the old drug dosage must be reduced slowly as the dosage of the new drug is increased. However carefully it is done, a real withdrawal is still experienced. Then the new drug must be given a chance — say over three months. When you are a teenager, life is very short and so is patience. Moreover, nobody had yet told me that epilepsy was chronic — and permanent. So I still expected miracles of instant control.

Since the onset of epilepsy, I have gradually become an amateur neurologist of necessity. From the inside I have learnt to recognize and label all the things that the neurologists, with their textbooks don't tell you, because they can't — they are not epileptics. In many ways I think it would be a great advantage for medical and nursing schools to admit people with such disorders as students, if not to practise on the public, then at least to carry out research. Only we can know exactly how we feel after a *grand mal*. Only we can say how long the recovery time really is, how much it affects our work and life, how much it affects our outlook. A neurologist who already knew the complexities of surviving as an epileptic would surely have an excellent starting point for his research.

Dr Ebeling was extremely quick at finding the root cause of any trouble I was having with the drugs. For a long time I was getting very drowsy in the afternoons and was liable to have a fit about nine o'clock at night.

'Good heavens!' he said irritably. 'You're supposed to be an intelligent girl. When do you take your pills?'

'Eight in the morning, noon and bed-time,' I answered belligerently. Defiance reached its peak during these consultations.

'Well, surely you don't have to be told that the pills should be spread out evenly through the day? Twenty-four hours in a day. Three lots of pills. Equals one lot to be taken every eight hours. Am I right? If your first dose is at 8 a.m., then your next dose shouldn't be until 4 p.m., or of course you'll get sleepy with a double dose of phenobarb in you. And of course you'll have a *grand mal* at night if the next lot of pills is too late!'

I nearly burst with anger — at myself, really, for not seeing that first. It was a simple and effective solution. For years I firmly believed that the pills must be taken exactly on time (my time!) or terrible things would happen to me. Later I discovered that the basic times (7 a.m., 3 p.m., and 11 p.m.) were fairly flexible as long as I swallowed the right amount each day. But leaving twelve hours between doses too often is just asking for trouble.

Between us, Dr Ebeling and I were able to reduce the number of *grand mals* considerably. But as soon as I became inquisitive about epilepsy, it was inevitable that I should get on to some bad information as well as good. I soon became aware that epilepsy had long been associated with mental illness, so I talked with Dr Ebeling about that also. He was not a psychiatrist and he strongly disapproved when I asked him if I needed one. I suppose he could see right through me and knew that I didn't need psychiatric help — although it would have been fascinating to find out what it was all about!

This brusque, matter-of-fact manner made me so indignant that I forgot to complain. It saved me from becoming a hypochondriac. Another doctor, more immediately sympathetic but less ultimately useful, might have included everything from neuralgia to pimples in the 'general symptoms' category. I would now be spending my life eagerly counting headaches, hot flushes, dizzy spells and nausea, and expecting my fingernails to fall out into the bargain. Thanks to Dr Ebeling, I confine all relevant factors to major and minor fits. Everything else I share in common with the rest of mankind.

After two years of experimentation with different combinations of drugs, a long trial-and-error process, the *grand mals* settled down into a once or twice a month pattern with occasional night fits as well. That's a pretty good record, really. A century ago someone like me would have been helpless at eighteen and more than likely dead at twenty.

But during this year I started having nightmares — watching myself being taken into hospital, lying in a large room (possibly an operating theatre) and then, paralysed with fear, watching myself die. A new and sinister aspect of the epilepsy was emerging — death-fear after a fit. It has stayed with me ever since.

Coming up from the bottom of the black ocean I can see the light again, but it can't prevent my grief or my immediate fear. I moan and cry, sobbing with terror, 'I don't want to die. Oh please don't let me die.' I can no more control this fear than I can control the fit itself. It is simply the next phase of a *grand mal* for me. Things around me may come back into view, but they still remain aloof, foreign, as if I were no longer a part of my surroundings. That fear and alienation embrace me completely for a few hours; then the defences return and my attitude to death is the same as yours.

Having a *grand mal* does feel rather like dying and starting to live again. This, plus the nightmares, slowly convinced me that I didn't have long to live. It is easy enough to dismiss such an idea now but, for a time, this dread took a strong hold of me. Questioning the doctors about my life-expectancy had drawn a blank. They were evasive. Naturally I interpreted this in the most gloomy way possible, and I think my mother had similar fears. I will never understand why such a crucial question was ignored and left unanswered. Possibly the doctors, knowing better, simply would not take it seriously. A bitterness, a hopelessness grew in me that year, and was precipitated by a new sort of fit that I began to discern — different from a *petit mal*. Before long I had christened it the 'Terror'.

When epileptics are tired, hungry, strained or just preoccupied, they are liable to small seizures. That's a good name for them because the brain seizes up just like a car engine that has run out of oil. The parts refuse to move and the brain refuses to continue thinking logically for several minutes. For me, this usually occurs when someone directs a question at me, or when my mind becomes totally absorbed in something like a wildflower in a hedge or the sight of someone else's beans sprouting beautifully when mine are showing no signs. It can be very embarrasing when an answer is required. I have never been able to think of a good excuse for totally ignoring someone's question, then asking him to repeat it but obviously having no idea what he is talking about. That is really just a *petit mal* — average recovery time, five minutes, during which the person has often stalked off in disgust. 'What's the matter with her? I just asked where she was up to and she looked quite blank!' People have every right to be indignant, but there's little I can do about it.

But the Terror is quite a different experience. More extensive, more dangerous even than a double *grand mal;* more terrifying because there are moments of consciousness in which I know what's happening, but there is nothing I can do to stop it snowballing into a thoroughly dangerous event. Neurologists call it 'temporal lobe epilepsy' (T L E for short).

It usually means that I'm overtired, or have forgotten my drugs. During this sort of seizure I feel as if there is a solid drill going right through the middle of my forehead and into my brain, twisting up the thought processes like a fork in a plate of spaghetti. It's not so much a pain as a most urgent event which may be fought for a little while, but eventually forces me to submit to it. Although I can continue what I am doing there is no guarantee that it is being done properly. For instance, I am likely to put out a whole line of washing without rinsing it even once, or remake the bed with only one sheet; or file an entire alphabet of cards into the Bs. I might say 'yes' when I should most assuredly have said 'no'; or put my father's address on my mother's letter; or just keep riding the bicycle around the block, oblivious of traffic lights, forgetting where I live. The instances, both funny and serious, are endless.

If all the warning signals are ignored, or, as is most often the case, if I'm simply not able to do anything about them, this continuing succession of small seizures sometimes explodes into a full-length T L E attack, which can last a whole afternoon. It may involve all my senses until I am caught up helplessly in a process very similar to the 'trip' described by people who take hard drugs.

Neurologists have described T L E as a form of automatism during which the patient involuntarily performs habitual actions and says ordinary phrases which, in context, can be quite meaningless. That is all they know about it. They obviously do not realize to what extent it can take over the patient. Never having seen myself in this kind of seizure, I can only describe T L E from the inside. The phases of oblivion are accented by moments of awareness during which I can almost watch myself, fascinated, against the hallucinatory background of a no-longer everyday life.

There was one bus ride which finally impressed upon me the fact that T L E must certainly be yet another manifestation of my little devil — and a more formidable one than a *grand mal*, because those around me cannot understand what is wrong, making my behaviour appear specially peculiar.

I was returning home after an afternoon full of warning signals of the Terror. The usual elements of hunger, fatigue and work interaction had started it, along with a new factor — loud, piped music in the bus going right through my head, making way for that inevitable drill. I felt pinned there and watched helplessly as the daylight faded and the lights of oncoming traffic glared at me. My ears started singing and my throat was dry. That bus ride became a singular event — all my senses were working at top pitch and all the messages they were conveying to the brain centre became twisted and distorted. The colour of the seats. The smell of stale fish and chips. Chocolate papers on the floor. The people. Just ordinary folk going home from work. I felt terribly involved with them, as if I knew them, their lives, joys, sorrows — all about them. How can I convey this concentrated instant? It was as if I was hovering over the whole scene and it telescoped into a split second, like a lightning flash imprinting itself upon my brain. I had a vision of the people in this bus, in this city, in this country, in the world, holding me fascinated. A lady wanted to get past me but I didn't understand and just stared at her. In a moment of consciousness I got terrified in case we'd gone past my stop. The driver was shouting, did I want to get out? What was he saying? Had I moved house? Near tears I rushed off the bus where he indicated (thank God for friendly bus-drivers). Someone threw my shopping out after me. And so it continued. . .

As short *petit mals* have decreased, these long T L E

attacks have increased enough to become a danger. What am I supposed to do about them? Stop whatever I am doing until it goes away? Fine – but first I have to recognize that something is wrong. That never happens until my brain un-jams and the spaghetti sorts itself out. That process can take several hours.

Most employers are unaware of this aspect of epilepsy. It is the more spectacular *grand mal* that they are worried about. Perhaps T L E is no more serious to them than absent-mindedness of plain laziness – both common enough human failings. It is easy to make up for an afternoon spent with the Terror. I just work doubly hard the next day. Well – if future employers are prepared to put up with absent-mindedness, why on earth should they mind if statistics showed that I might have one fit in a year during working hours?

One of the possible side-effects of epilepsy, as with any condition that tends to set the patient apart from the rest of mankind for any length of time, is paranoia – plain old persecution complex. It is all very easy for me to say that now, as a cool observation. But for a good eight years at least, my little world was continually coming to a sad end and I cut myself off from people rather than take a chance on being hurt. Either everybody hated me, or I hated everybody, or else life was generally unbearable. It would have been so nice if somebody had told me that this attitude was actually a symptom, half of which was imagined and the rest being an aggravated result of said imaginings. Once you know about something it is so much easier to deal with.

But nobody told me about paranoia and so my memory of the following few years, if not scrupulously screened, is one of unrelieved misery. I would sit in my room and listen to Peter, Paul and Mary singing the American folksong, *Old Coat*. They were singing straight at me.

Like some ragged owlet,
With its wings expanded,
Nailed to some garden gate or hoarding.
Thus will I by some men
All my life be branded . . . .
Never hurted none this side of Jordan.

Well — it all fitted. Didn't it? I certainly looked ragged enough; and I was beginning to find out what it meant to be branded. That's the interpretation that I managed to put on every little episode in my first job.

A busy general hospital is a happy and sociable place to work in. With so many people on the non-medical staff, there is usually at least one small group with whom one can feel an affinity. But my extremely mixed attitudes were leading to problems and, sometimes, appalling scenes. I had never met such a variety of people in all my life and I had no idea how to handle the most ordinary situation. I was utterly confounded when the dark-room attendant offered to buy me tea and a bun. Whenever one of the radiographers had a bad day and came over to the developing machine and wept when she saw that she had mismanaged a difficult X-ray for the third time, I was like Chicken Licken and thought the sky was falling in.

There was one grand old doctor who terrified all the radiographers. She was an absolute perfectionist. A woman in a man's world, she had to struggle extra hard to retain her position, and her opinion was widely respected. She was small with bowed shoulders, a sharp tongue and white corkscrew curls. She reminded me, on the days when her tongue was not directed at me, of Miss Marple. It was usually she who sent the young trainee radiographers back to their machines with a metaphorical cuff on the ear and a certainty that their next attempts would be even worse.

Initially I made friends because the kind-hearted radiographers were interested in my planned university career. But I had not learned how to reinforce friendships so I was soon at loggerheads with most of the staff, feeling socially inferior and intellectually superior.

Soon the university gambit began to wear thin and I tried another way — by telling people in the strictest confidence about my 'grave disability', stressing (and exaggerating) the difficult and even hopeless prospects it gave me. But crocodile tears are a pretty useless basis for friendship, too. There my resources and imagination ended.

For the whole of that year, while I was working at the hospital, I spent the evenings shut in my room, teaching myself classical music and making an elaborate tapestry — hardly an atmosphere to foster optimism or self-help. I wasn't even trying to learn the practicalities of being master of my own destiny. What was the point — if I had no destiny to be master of? But there was really no need to cut myself off from life — it was a bad mistake. It was carrying martyrdom to extremes. I was seventeen.

Desiderata says, 'Many fears are born of fatigue and loneliness . . . .' Exactly. I was probably no more tired than anyone else in their first year at work. But I was desperately lonely. Hence the death-fear. It was all very well to be physically daring. That is the easiest kind of courage. I had no moral courage whatsoever. Somehow I managed to forget the tea and buns offered by the young man in the X-ray darkroom. If someone was having a bad day, my supersensitivity blew up small incidents into a war directed straight at me. I would run and hide behind my grand excuse, thinking everyone mean and hostile. ('Stop the world, I wanna get off. Nobody loves me, everybody hates me — I think I'll go and eat worms'). A permanent sulk doesn't exactly invite people to renew their acquaintance. Inevitable result — utter misery and a huge chip on the shoulder. I forgot how to smile.

It was about this time that I discovered the magnetism of High Anglicanism: the lure of dim churches, the smell of incense, the plainsong and canticles, the feeling of sanctuary and belonging. St Peter's in Melbourne is directly across the street from St Pat's, the Roman Catholic cathedral. In those days we still had those gorgeous old green trams with polished, wooden seats, which would cruise along the middle of the road at a maximum speed of twenty-five miles per hour, to the delight of tourists and small boys, and to the chagrin of motorists. These trams went past St Peter's and were part of the joy of going there.

St Peter's could scarcely be called a Church of England at all. It had an altar full of crucifixes, numerous statues of Mary and the smell of incense — all the natural colour of the Roman Church. The priests were called 'Father' and were celibate. There was even reputed to be a tunnel under the street for the exchange of altar boys! All this high church ritual is more or less permitted within the Anglican constitution and it satisfied the spiritual needs of many of the people worshipping there at the time. But there was also a collection of loners like myself, all hoping to bury their various hangups in the all-encompassing ceremonial of the church. There was even provision for confession.

For those brought up in the ways of the Roman Catholic church, all these things are accepted as a normal part of religion. But to be attracted to a church simply because of all the trappings rather than the central theme is definitely unhealthy and liable to lead to all sorts of confusion. In my mind I began to mix up sin, guilt, epilepsy, redemption, the Holy Spirit and the Chosen of God, until my vision of self grew even more distorted. Nobody tried to enlighten me; it was not a communicative church community. There was a tea held after evensong where I used to sit and look hopeful, occasionally speaking about the weather to a pimply youth.

Apart from burying myself in religion, I buried myself in books. The train journey took about half an hour each way into the city of Melbourne, plus about a quarter of an hour on the tram out to the hospital, depending on the traffic. Huge tomes, I chose, to transport me far away into other times, other countries and other lives. And so,

I made a great find — but it was to prove a mixed blessing in my exaggerated state of mind.

In general, authors don't seem to use epilepsy in their attempt to put on paper the great human condition. Purely by chance, I read *The Idiot,* by Dostoevsky. Prince Mishkin, the hero of this story, remains the most beautiful representation of an epileptic in all literature. Authors are not generally willing to write about something of which they understand little. But Dostoevsky himself was an epileptic, having such frequent and serious *grand mals* that his work was often affected.

The Idiot contains many long and detailed descriptions which only one of us could write; from the smallest preoccupation with an object and enforced vagueness to the whole sequence of a *grand mal*. Dostoevsky does not spare his gentle, saintly idiot, but loves his hero none the less. Written in 1869, this novel probably shows the fate of many epileptics before the discovery of adequate anti-convulsant drugs. After much treatment designed to get him to a fairly normal state, Mishkin is suddenly launched into the world. Here his trusting innocence and passion for truth lead him into such serious trouble that he becomes unbearably confused and reverts to his former condition. Mishkin's struggles in high society are related from the prince's own point of view, which is that either everyone else is mad or he is — and the reader may often get the impression that Mishkin is the only sane person in his small circle! The book shows the curiosity, affection and even forgiveness of the people Mishkin encounters during his brief stay in the world of Russian wealth. He is a revelation to them and he can laugh at himself with them, too. All possible reactions to his affliction are represented — that he is simple or else very clever, that he is sick and therefore bad, that he uses his illness, and that he is a saint. I recognized so much of myself in Mishkin — from the broken chains of ideas to intensity of experience and the determination not to hide.

There was no question about Russian society not accepting Mishkin. They were all anxious to meet him and very curious as to how he would look and act: Does he wave his arms? Does he fall down frequently? Must he wear a napkin all the time? (presumably he dribbled.) But on meeting and talking with Mishkin, they decided he is perhaps not so odd after all — quite acceptable, in fact. Mishkin himself is not afraid or ashamed of being an epileptic. People question him eagerly about the whole process of his illness and he answers diffidently but without dissimulation. Through Mishkin, the author describes all the essential things that happen to epileptics even today: *petit mal* in the middle of a long story; attacks of the Terror during which he does things automatically and without logical sequence; a real epileptic *grand mal* when the horrified onlookers hear his wild scream 'as if a spirit were tearing him apart', see his distorted face and presume that he must be in terrible agony. He also describes Mishkin's 'beatific moments' — times of intense joy and peace and illumination which may happen just before a *grand mal.*

Reading this book made me eternally grateful for twentieth-century medicine. A hundred years ago the rich would be given spartan treatment of cold-water baths and gymnastics along with careful diet and a regulated life. The poor were at the mercy of circumstances until they injured themselves fatally. Also, it was generally agreed that epileptics could not marry. Many laws were passed concerning this in Europe alone, and some have still not been repealed, although they are universally ignored. Mishkin admits that, owing to his illness, he 'knew nothing of women'. Mishkin is naive, ingenuous, extremely anxious to please and appears simple because his speech is not equal to his ideas, as I was soon to discover, also. He is often insufferably sad, 'lost in wonder and uneasiness', a fair description of what T L E feels like.

In the days of Dostoevky, it was a brave man who suffered from epilepsy and yet decided to live in society and maintain as much independence as possible. But how different are our circumstances now! And how I wish other people would realize it! It was to be many years before I could glean a constructive ideology from this great book. The first time that I read it, it gave only a rationale for bitterness, for setting myself apart and for withdrawing from society. By the end of my first year outside school, I had cut myself off from all channels of communication, sources of mutual confidence and friendships. Rarely speaking to the family on anything but the most mundane matters, my voluntary separation was complete. Not a healthy situation. But there was nobody else to blame.

6

Surely when you are so very low things can only get better?
At least I thought so — with a complete break from the
hospital job and a new start, everything would be different. On the night before my first day at university, I lay
on the back lawn looking at the glorious, starry sky, and
resolving to do nothing but study for three years, I believed the world was at my feet.

At that time, Melbourne University outshone its only
other rival among the universties in Victoria. They served
about two million people. There were 14,000 students
enrolled in 1966, doing every imaginable (orthodox)
course. In spite of being cramped by the old houses of
Parkville, the City, and the Melbourne General Cemetery,
the facilities were excellent, with plenty of sports areas
and a large student union complex. 'The Caf' was the meeting place for all and sundry, and a huge endowed library
provided adequate space for those who wanted to work.
There was no student unrest, although a few years later,
an infiltrator called 'The Wizard' came to power, so the
usual succession of strikes and sit-ins cropped up. In fact
it was a lively, interesting place with plenty of opportuni-
ties for every variety of person.

The first week of university was one long entertainment
put on for us, the Freshers. Older students gave us a Freshers'
breakfast of weak tea, cold toast and rubberized fried
eggs; they themselves were dressed in absurd pyjamas and
voluptuous nightdresses. The entire week was so hot that
we all ended up, fully clad, under the lawn sprinklers by
three o'clock every afternoon. All the clubs and societies
courted us with displays (their minds principally on sub-
scription fees) and there were the more sober affairs of

welcome speeches and the arrangement of classes. It took over two hours to make the actual enrolment; we had to complete at least thirty cards or forms containing our personal and subject details. This particular young woman, with all her supposed handicaps and background disadvantages, had actually made it, on her own merits, to the best university in Australia. That was quite a feat. I had a sort of vision of myself as the extra-long-suffering saintly blue-stocking genius of all time.

I joined the gym club (on, the joys of trampolining — yet another forbidden form of physical defiance) and, of course, the Anglican Society. Fortunately, or so I thought, this society was High Church in its leaning. The president was a brilliant history honours student who later became a Jesuit priest. The secretary was a brilliant, highly strung girl, who showed some benevolent interest in me. Like the president she was also eccentric — her platform was equality for women within the church and she took great pride in being the altar boy at our weekly communion services. She could also sing. She, the president and the priest could hold the floor for hours on the subject of church policy with great learning, much jargon and no apparent feeling whatsoever. Between them they fabricated a beautiful and elaborate cassock with nothing inside it. I admired them tremendously.

If trampolining was not exactly advisable, my choice of subjects was a further stroke of defiance. All right, I said, if they're not going to let me be anything when I have finished, I will do a course which would confound anyone to find a career to follow it. And I did. Doing a double major in the History and Philosophy of Science was very interesting, possibly improving and of no benefit whatsoever to the community who were paying for it.

Within a few months my recurring persecution complex had reduced the glorious vision of the epileptic-who-made- it to a farce. I had been naive to expect that simply being at university would solve all my relationship-acceptance problems. I would sit in biology lectures, and in between drawing pictures of platyhelminthes or dicotyledons, I would look around at everyone else and decide that I was, definitely, the second plainest girl there.

There was so much to enjoy — if only I could have put aside my fears and defences to enjoy it. English lectures, for instance, were a reverential experience. Professor Maxwell should have been retired, but he could not resist the temptation to come and lecture to us first-years on the subject of Border ballads. In his black gown, shiny and tattered with age, he would stand at the rostrum and recite his favourite ballads by heart, often taking out a well-used white handkerchief into which he would blow a long, mournful note. Then, wiping each eye behind his glasses he would continue:

> '*O why does thy hand sae drap wie blude,*
> *Edward, Edward . . . .*'

There was not a whisper from any of the five hundred or so in the biggest lecture hall on the campus. No paper darts. No Jaffas (chocolate balls with orange coating) rolling down the steps from top to bottom. Just the silence of respect.

The times in between lectures grew to have a nightmarish quality for me. Nobody walked around the university grounds alone; nobody sunbaked alone under the gums outside the library, except me. I was always a hit with people in the beginning. Perhaps my impulsiveness and recklessness were mistaken for warmth and courage. But friendships are cemented by respect — and I had no cement. In desperation, I would always reveal my secret to new acquaintances, and wait for a reaction. There always was one: a spark of new interest, a glimmer of admiration. But honestly, what did I expect them to do. Jump up and down? Ask me to marry them on the spot? Swear everlasting friendship? Tell me how lovely I was? God knows. And when the spark died, there was I, left disillusioned; I had played my last card and still lost the game.

The long, green galley-slips of examination papers were unrolled over three weeks of intense heat, answered with moderate ease, and rolled up again. I might have passed that sort of test with no trouble, but exams were secondary in importance to the harder tests of socialization. I had failed that part of life miserably. I could not understand why or what I was doing wrong. It just had not worked. Very early on I wrote:

> *I am rejected.*
> *I felt it come upon me like a revelation*
> *And I said it aloud, surprised when*
> *After they had gone, I was alone . . .*
> *No more was I to be invited*
> *Or even accepted by them*
> *To walk, to dine, to sit and discuss*
> *They did not want the special something that was me*
> *There — a part of their unity.*

Three years later, just before graduation, you can see how far I'd got:

> *I guess now, I leave this place*
> *As lonely as the day I entered it.*
> *But it was not for nothing, all this.*
> *O, no. I got something from it — didn't I?*
> *Yeah — a wider realization of what it is*
> *To be condemned to loneliness . . .*
> *So, then. I am rejected.*

Perhaps if I had understood more of the nature of epilepsy, I might have made a more valiant fight. But in the absence of facts, imagination is bound to run riot. I began to compare myself to all sorts of things. In particular, I would extrapolate from the folksong until I became a baby owl in a barn, all scruffy and uncertain, flapping about in the dark, hooting miserably and bumping into unknown objects. Discovering that I had no friends and no social life, I was prepared to blame it all on epilepsy. Epilepsy was changing my personality. Epilepsy was ruining my life. Thus fighting and flapping blindly away, I had overlooked the likelihood that it could not have been very different. From childhood, I was heading towards being a hermit anyway.

Quite simply, all faith in my own intuition and judgement had been shattered. That left me with everyone else's standards to live up to. Having one person's mind and another's body just doesn't work. I valued myself even less than I thought everyone else did.

The Secretary of the Anglican Society decided in her wisdom that I had a special cross for which I should be really thankful. It was a great favour of God to be possessed by a spirit because it meant that I was being given extra trials to endure. And I believed her! She did one good thing for me — she persuaded me to leave the constraints of home and go to live in one of the women's colleges. For better or worse, I went.

There is a popular old wives' tale — 'third time lucky'. The move to college would have been the third time that I had made a major new start — with a new set of people in a new set of surroundings. Surely this time I would uncover the clue to social success? There was, certainly, a respite from all the directionless struggling. At least I belonged there.

Ours was the oldest established women's college in Victoria. Australia was not quite ready to mix its sexes, even at university level. But rules were not so terribly strict and we all had keys to the main door so we could come and go at leisure. We wore gowns for formal dinners but there were no other compulsions. In the first week of term there was the freshers' exam, which I failed, not knowing the definition of the Sheepwalk (path in front of the adjacent men's college) or the Bulpaddock (place where men now played football, but where a bull used to graze during the war — the college war effort!); nor the names of the three college cats; nor the difference, other than biological, between Mrs Dodds and Mr Sainty (cook and gardener). However, I made up for the appalling lack of general knowledge by participating successfully in the Freshers' mystery race. In this we were all given a long poem with many obscure references to things and/or people which had to be collected. Then we were sent out in pairs and expected to bring back as many of the things (however we interpreted them), as possible in one afternoon. One of the items was a Micksmaster which really meant the Warden of the Roman Catholic men's college. But my partner and I found a genuine non-English speaking Italian bricklayer and brought him back, complete with his cement mixer (of which the brand name was something like 'Mixmaster'). For our efforts we received a 6d each as a reward for initiative and ingenuity; the puzzled Italian only received half a pint of Melbourne bitter.

In that first year at college I lived in the ground floor and spent most of my nights letting in freshers who had come back late or older girls who had forgotten their keys. We were a select little group, just four of us opposite the music rooms; the final movement of Schumann's Piano Concerto is stamped indelibly on my brain. We held regular coffee parties, often inviting other second-years from the first floor. One of them I discovered to be an unknown distant cousin from the Queensland branch of our ubiquitous, pioneering family.

There were many friends to be made and interests to be followed. Somebody even discovered I could sing. Once they had managed to convince me of the fact, they could not stop me singing. I bought a guitar and started singing along with all my folk records, without mercy to my neighbours. It grew into a positive joy and I joined the college choir. My voice was (perhaps fortunately) not strong, having been asleep for eighteen years. But what a revelation! There is an example of just how bad my inhibitions had become. It took someone a lot of arguing to persuade me that I had inherited the voice which I ought to have anyway with so much music on both sides of the family.

I went for an unprecedented nine months without a *grand mal* during the day. There were numerous night fits, though, as proved by my waking up with a wet pillow, a bitten tongue and a swollen cheek every few weeks. My head felt as if it was floating for most of the day, but at least night fits were much easier to dismiss to myself than a *grand mal* in public. I began to stop fighting the inevitability of my lot as an epileptic, began to accept the fact. I even made some positive moves towards trying to live alongside it instead of against it.

My harum-scarum spirit had gravitated naturally towards a group of daredevil second-years, who would be off on some escapade at a moment's notice. One night they might go on a 'poppy expedition' to steal flowers from the beautiful university gardens — roses and camellias, pansies and sweet williams — for their own rooms. Another day several of them might suddenly be off to the surf beaches beyond Geelong or perhaps the blue ranges north of Melbourne, just to quench their thirst for escape and freedom for a short while. If I was to go with them, it would be inconvenient, to say the least, if I kept saying, 'Can you just hold on a minute while I go and get my pills?' So I made a tiny, strong pill-bag out of linen, embroidered it with a rose, secured it with press-studs and hung it around my neck. It would hold a day's worth of pills and it became my close friend and ally.

Nobody had seen me have a *grand mal* at work, or during my university years. The epilepsy seemed to have evened out into a pattern of night fits plus a liberal sprinkling of the Terror — T L E. Once attacks have become stabilized there is no real need to keep going to a specialist, having E E Gs or checkups. There is, at present, nothing more that can be done. Initially I was angry and bitter that Dr Ebeling would not try to 'do something' for me; eventually I realized that I was enjoying the freedom of forgetting completely, for long periods at a time, that I could be considered in any way special or different. The mere fact of going to the out-patient's clinic so often had been enough to perpetuate this idea. It had intruded into my life. But it had now been established that the cause of the fits was neither a brain tumour, nor physical or even chemical deficiencies. The experiments with all the possible combinations of drugs had been completed. Now I could simply settle down to a life of drug-taking; hence the little pill-bag. No doses must be forgotten, for if I miss one, I can expect a *grand mal* within two days. Strangely enough, the regular taking of pills is not a constant reminder of disability, not in the same way, at least as wearing an identification bracelet. It is just like someone knowing that they take saccharin in their tea or coffee, without immediately associating it with the fact that they are overweight or have a tendency to heart disease.

The close alliance with the college daredevils was, admittedly, just a continuation of my defiance of all the walls which had been set around me from the age of fifteen. But at last I found a rationale to support this attitude, so noticeably at odds with all common sense. It was not going to be enough for me that I just stay alive with the help of a cupboard full of pills. I was determined to experience everything, particularly those activities from which I was specifically barred. And my guiding star in this enterprise would be — a cockroach!

In my literary wanderings I had finally come across Archy, the philosophical cockroach, and Mehitabel his friend, the cat who had known better days. Don Marquis, in fact. Now Archy understands a lot about life and is willing to learn from even the most unlikely source. In this way he had discovered one view of living from another friendship of his, brief though it was. He met a moth who would come into the office, attracted by the lamp. This moth adored light with his whole soul and he yearned to be part of the light, even though he knew it was very dangerous — as many beautiful and moving things are. Archy asked him why he kept flying at the flame when it was courting death. The moth replied that he would prefer to live briefly and fully, worshipping the thing that he loved so much, rather than skulk in the dark, only half living and preserving himself from the very centre of his existence. One day the moth flew too close to the flame and was engulfed. One moment of absolute ecstasy, when moth and flame were one, then — extinguished. Archy respected the moth's choice, although he thought it unlikely that he would ever go to such lengths to seek ecstasy.

A young epileptic must also make choices, life-and-death choices sometimes, between his own safety and doing the sort of thing that most people do without even considering danger. It can be hard and it can lead to a lot of frustration unless the decisions are carefully handled and adequate substitutes are found. In my second year at university I began throwing my lot in with Archy's mothy friend, regardless of other people's concern, and flagrantly breaking all the most elementary rules for people with epilepsy. I was desperately determined to enjoy myself, and to hell with the cost. My little devil could do his worst and see how much I cared. But, I had also been assigned a very efficient guardian angel.

The university medical officer had advised me to apply for 'special consideration' during the examinations, in case of a fit. This would almost certainly mean that my paper would be marked separately, alongside all those who asked for consideration because of nervous breakdowns, difficulties in home life or with marriage partners, those who had all manner of medical certificates — in other words, my work would not be considered on its own merits. How would I know if I was really any good at the subject? But if I did not apply, and I had a fit during an examination, the officer said it would be a whole year's work gone west. So I compromised, and made an application which was *only* to be considered in the case of a *grand mal* before or during an exam. Actually I never believed for a minute that any such thing could happen. Never had I had a fit during a time of stress. This application was only a weakness, a giving in to other people's ideas about epilepsy.

While awaiting the exam results, the hard core of the college daredevils (including myself) went cherry-picking in the mountains. There was nothing so exhilarating as standing at the top of a ladder singing 'Hey Jude' into the crystal-clear air and (incidentally) filling our boxes with cherries. They were homemade inventions, those boxes — about ten inches square with a long belt of real leather which was slung around the waist and attached to the other side of the picking box by a bent nail. These we would periodically empty into the bigger fruit boxes. A good picker would get through thirty cases a day but I thought eleven was fairly good. It was a long day, twelve hours, starting at 7 a.m. We college girls lived in a one-room shanty up by the cool store, the big shed where fruit was stored for any length of time at a fairly cold temperature. There were four of us on two iron beds with a wooden toilet out the back. We had to bang the seat before using this primitive contrivance, in the hopes that brown snakes and the deadly red-backed spiders would leave us alone for a few minutes.

From the cherry orchards we could see, on a clear day, right across to the year-round snow atop Mt Donna Buang. My mother would have had nightmares seeing me balance on top of those ladders. I always volunteered to do the tree-middle as well — fewer cherries of course, but there was the added joy of standing precariously with my feet hooked around two branches while the wind shook the dark leaves, and often me as well. What if . . .? But it didn't and my neck remained intact.

Every day we extravagantly ordered a newspaper because the university results would be published in all the dailies just around Christmas time. I passed the second year well — two passes and two honours — which meant I could return to college and expect a good room. The living allowance from the Commonwealth Scholarship was paying for it, too — just. In my final year I had a beautiful room on the top floor of the old college where I wrote essays late into the night and only stopped when I heard the old milk-horse shaking the churns as he trotted down the lane around 3 a.m.

All of the college daredevils returned as well, some as exalted fourth-years and most as highly honoured third-years. But we were not to be content with short escapades this year. We required a vehicle. I seemed to be the only one of our small circle with any spare money so I bought a very cheap, very ancient car, a Vauxhall Six, for the use of friends. (I soon discovered that I was to be precluded from driving, on medical grounds.) This car was ever so tall compared with the more modern Holdens, Fords and Morrises, and very narrow as well — quite a lady — so we named her Harriett (the Chariot).

Harriett took us on many long ventures all over Victoria, especially camping expeditions in the bush. She came to an untimely end one dark and moonless night on the Murray Valley Highway (an unmade road with a town every twenty or thirty miles) when she turned a bend and met a cow. It was a large, black, Poll-Friesian cross who should not have been there at all. The cow had the good manners to get up off the road and walk into the marsh where she died after making horrible gurgling noises for an hour or two. As for the three of us in the car, we were quite stranded. Not a soul had passed us in over an hour; no phone or house was likely to be within twenty miles, let along a policeman. Finally, a drunk lurched towards us in a beat-up Holden, having crossed the border from New South Wales (where there were civilized closing hours) and managed to find a police station and a town for us.

That was not exactly the end of Harriet but it proved ultimately fatal. Harriett was going to cost us $150 to repair. We all raised money by giving private tutorials to struggling first-year students, as we were then in third year. My gentleman student was quite a character. He had been recommended to me by the small History and Philosophy of Science department and was a Hungarian immigrant (a mature student trying to gain a Melbourne Bachelor of Arts in order to return to his former profession of teaching). While I was busy explaining the Aristotelian world view and the Ptolemaic Universe, he plied me with herb teas which he brought in small medicine bottles, eventually admitting that they were Hungarian peasant aphrodisiac recipes. We used to try to analyse them but were careful to pour them down the sink. He passed too!

Harriett was never herself again and she just exploded on her way down the Geelong road, one blastingly hot summer's day. We never found her oil cap, and her entire engine was split across. Dear Harriett — at least she died in a blaze of glory.

7

College days were often happy. But we were only continuing our adolescence there and life was very sheltered. Many of us had still not discovered who we were. So it was also a very stormy time, full of tears and tantrums, broken friendships and loves, the discovery of drunkenness and even suicide.

Unfortunately my great expectations for a major self-transformation went unfulfilled. Third time lucky was not really holding water, after all. The magic formula for friendship and the expectancy of love were still eluding me. Even in that huge beehive of people I remained basically alone despite my dubious reputation with the daredevils. It is true that they were prepared to include me at any time, and their friendship was certainly valuable. They were not the socialite types — people with rich daddies and smart clothes — nor were they the sensible, serious plodders who studied around the clock. Rather, this little circle of people were a bit unusual, *avant-garde*, used to having eyebrows slightly raised when they passed. Outsiders saw them as clever, especially with words. They were also experimenting with feelings, and, most importantly for me, they respected individuals just as they were, without trying or even wanting to change them.

On good days I was glad of their welcome and willing to join in their escapades. On bad days I could not even open my door, but sat inside my shell, wrote 'rejection' poetry and thought seriously of seeing a trick cyclist. In reality, these good and bad days were something I experienced in common with half the world population — a simple, biological rhythm. But I couldn't accept that — oh no, I was special; I was different.

What exactly went wrong that year? How could it possibly have turned out to be the most traumatic succession of miseries that life had yet presented me with? I was continually at odds with the college environment, swimming desperately against the stream.

'Are you fighting the whole world?' asked Joan, one of my longest-suffering friends.

'Yes,' I replied, in all seriousness.

She tried to calm me down by telling me the story of the Wind and the Sun. She was an excellent storyteller, and later became a highly successful English and drama teacher.

The Wind and the Sun decided to have a competition to see who was the strongest.

'Okay,' said the Wind, positive that he would win, 'See that man walking along the road? Well, I reckon I can get his coat off quicker than you. It is a bet?'

The Sun smiled and nodded.

'Cor!' thought the Wind. 'That old Sun hasn't a chance — it's hardly worth the effort.' Nevertheless, he blew hard down the road and set the man's coat flapping. Laughing, the Wind turned back and swooped at the man whose coat was half off his back already. 'It's in the bag,' said the Wind. He turned around and blew his hardest. But the man had got wise — he pulled his coat closely about him and no amount of blowing would move the coat. The Wind was winded.

'Okay, you try,' he said sulkily to the Sun. All she did was to beam warmly down on the man. Muttering something rude about "Changeable weather in this part of the world", he became so hot, the sweat beading on his forehead, that he just sat right down and took his coat off. The Sun had won.

According to Joan I was that man and the wind was all the buffeting I had received, even if a lot of it was all my own fault. The coat was obviously my wrong-headedness. Perhaps now it was time for some gentle warmth to take the chill off my undeveloped little person, bristling like a hedgehog with defences. But I was literally refusing to

79

'let the sunshine in'. Even my mother had given up her tears and prayers, knowing that I was determined to tread my own suicidal path to personal destruction.

I grew more frozen, badly needing someone to put an arm around me and say, 'Don't worry. It'll be okay. We love you anyway. Stop fighting so hard — you're not a frog in a bowl of milk!' A few friends did manage to melt me a little, to stop me going so fast in the wrong direction. But always I had this lever over people — that I was an epileptic and therefore (presumably) they should feel sorry for me and be nice to me. This is the single most stupid, most dangerous attitude that epileptics can have about themselves and their disability. It causes an immediate over-sympathetic, over-protective reaction in people, nearly always followed sooner or later by an equally strong counter-reaction against the epileptic. It is so easy for us to expect a yard from people who believe that it may be reasonable to give an inch, but think it not in the interests of any disabled person to give too much leeway. I had now got to the stage of unreasonable expectations.

Finally, Joan suggested that a psychiatrist might be able to help this unhappy trend. A few years earlier, the exasperated Dr Ebeling had finally let me go to the clinic psychiatrist. After one session it must have been obvious to this man that I was just relating what I thought he should be interested in; I was wasting his time. Dr Ebeling's strictly self-help philosophy was vindicated. But by third-year university, I was becoming really frightened of where it was all leading. At the age of twenty, there was not a single person who I could happily call 'friend'. I had come to believe that there was something terribly basic that I was doing wrong at the beginning of a possible friendship. The blue exercise book full of rejection poetry becomes violet with misery.

> . . . How very futile is my attempt
> To communicate, or become one of them
> Because there is something elementary,

Well before the long, gay time
That severs me, shuts me out,
It says firmly, 'No'. When a certain point is
reached. No. Nor further . . . .

Finally, thoroughly convinced that I was indeed in need of help, I made an appointment to see a private trick cyclist, using up half of my holiday earnings. This is a trap that many epileptics and others with chronic diseases are liable to fall into. To all these people I recommend the Ebeling do-it-yourself treatment. Just because you have a scar on your brain doesn't mean that you can kid yourself into thinking that you're mentally unstable. It simply doesn't follow. If you are really in a bad way it might be better to consult a minister and his wife whose sincerity you respect. They can be amazingly realistic and tell you what they think in no uncertain terms.

My man was youngish, pale with dark hair and a bit too much flab. He leaned back in his confortable chair and chewed a pencil while I poured out all my story. The blank paper in front of him remained blank. The sun was shining hotly through his Collins Street venetian blinds. About three quarters of an hour later I suddenly stopped. He had not said a single word. I dried up. Patiently he waited for me to go on, not even begging me to continue. He looked just a little bored, probably was not even listening and certainly had not heard anything worth recording. I had one of my flashes of vision. This time I saw myself, looking very small and being very trivial. There was nothing wrong with me that could not be put right with a bit of will-power — or tolerance, for that matter. The man must have been good, I conclude, for I never went back again. Ever since, at any really bad time when I am considering being analysed, the memory of that session is enough to put me off. Freud can carry on without me.

8

Amazingly, I never seriously thought about what I would do after this degree. Whether it was apathy or serenity, I closed my mind to the problem. Everyone else from college either had serious partners whom they planned to marry or else had their careers fairly well mapped out. I had no boyfriends and only a few immature crushes to my score, being hopelessly socially inept and frankly frightened of being with more than one person at a time. Heaven knows what perversity, in the shape of the careers officer, urged me to train for teaching. That is the last sort of person who should go into a classroom of noisy school-children, intending to control them. However, I passed the final examinations, enrolled for Dip Ed. and moved out of college.

Carlton, the square mile of intensive housing which lies due north of the City of Melbourne precinct, is the most important source of accommodation for anybody connected with the large university. Many of the streets are wide with central built-up strips of grass and plane trees. Some of the houses have been restored to their pure-white, Victorian glory — and many more have been condemned as unfit for human habitation. It is to the latter that most of the post-graduate students go. That way they are able to work in the library or laboratories until all hours. Also they can feel a permanent part of this great, all-enveloping university complex and participate fully in the numerous activities. So it was in Carlton that I chose to live during my year of teacher-training.

I found a condemned terrace house very close to the university and shared it with five other assorted students.

My room was tiny — a veritable broom-cupboard, with just enough room for a bed, a table and a wardrobe — but no chance of swinging a cat. The window was about eight feet away from that of an artist in the next house (assorted students also). He was perfecting a method of abstract art using a narrow paint roller all over the canvas and ending with a large red or green gummed paper spot. They had titles like 'Emergence' and 'Discovery'; or (with two spots) 'Reunion'. He is probably famous now. At other times he had models in his bedroom, often forgetting to draw the curtains while he drew studies of the small of their backs. His spare time was spent writing his own defence for the ensuing court case in which he would be tried as a pacifist for evading conscription. Many great works were being used in this thesis, beginning with the Bible and Aristotle, and ending with Karl Marx and the Beatles. If his plea failed he faced two years' imprisonment with hard labour. The government had no time for pacifists during the sixties. Bright brown eyes, a tousled red head and bushy beard completed the picture. We would spend many a warm night solving the world's problems across eight feet of air, to the annoyance of anybody who wanted to sleep or study.

My only view, apart from his bedroom, was a huge oak tree, probably planted when the houses were built. I can still remember the shape of its bare twigs during our short winter, when the street lights shone right through them, magnifying the raindrops which hung from each nodule. I must have spent hundreds of hours just staring at that light, trying to understand the meaning of life and my current situation.

In the next house was also a beautiful girl with long fair hair that she could sit on, who spoke perfect BBC English and cooked hair-raising Latvian curries which I occasionally tried, but found it necessary to eat more fruit salad than curry. A most striking character in our house was Sean, an Irishman well over six feet tall, who I suspected of being as Australian as the rest of us. He and his parents were trying to put him through an Honours

Physics degree and he rather enjoyed his extreme depriva-
tion. He had heavy black hair, glittering black eyes set in
a chalk-white face, and long, pale fingers. He only ate when
he remembered to and my most lasting impression of Sean
is seeing him in the kitchen, searching for a can opener
for his daily tin of beans; he then ate the beans slowly and
deliberately from the tin with a spoon, if he could find
one. All the while his large, smouldering eyes would look
silently and reproachfully at the rest of us indulging in such
luxuries as cheese-on-toast or fried eggs, with an occasional
sausage.

Sean and I were in love — for a few weeks. It was a wonderful revelation to me, this love, and all too short but,
nevertheless, in it I found a sort of salvation, that held me
up and revivified my all-time low self-respect. It was a miracle, in a way. But soon he was off, after more interesting
pursuits. Sean was a year or two younger, and he was just
as interested in getting drunk as in putting himself out for
a girl.

It was in May, two months after I joined that house,
that my own graduation ceremony was held. For the first
time I was permitted to wear a gown with its sleeves slit,
but we were not required to wear mortar-boards for
ordinary degrees. There were too many of us and the hire
firms could not cope. Nobody was likely to buy one of those
absurd, flat hats with a tassel for everyday wear. After
the usual speeches I received a Bachelor of Arts degree,
shaking the revered hand of Sir Robert Menzies.

In general, festivities or solemn occasions like this were a
problem within the family. Whichever parent I decided
to spend Christmas or Easter with, the other would be
indignant. For some years I had taken to spending Christmas in Geelong with another family. But on the day I
graduated both my mother and my father came to watch
the ceremony. One sat upstairs while the other sat down-
stairs. They did not meet.

Many people's personal experience will prove that being
the child of divorced parents is not really so tragic and

damning as is often thought. Most of us survive. Admittedly I was lucky, having regular access to my father and brothers, and never going near a children's home, foster parent, court of access or social worker. It was silly for me to write myself off on those grounds; there was no earthly reason why I should not have a normal adult life, as the long and happy marriages of the other five children in the family prove. But at twenty-one I raged against my parents, putting much of the blame on them for everything that had (or had not) happened to me, including becoming an epileptic. But I was to discover that I had no right to lay such blame, any more than the parents of an epileptic should ever feel guilty for their child's disability.

It was by pure chance that I happened across a chapter on epileptic children as extra reading for one of the subjects in Dip Ed. What I found out was that epilepsy itself cannot be inherited. What we get by way of inheritance is a certain sort of threshold for epilepsy. Most people have all kinds of accidents from being dropped on the stairs when they are babies to major car accidents later on, yet they emerge without lasting damage. This is because most people have what neurologists call a higher threshold for epilepsy. Their brain function is less liable to electrical disturbance. Other people have a lower threshold. Given that they already have a brain lesion, caused by a head injury or a difficult birth, plus serveral other factors all converging on them at once (rage, grief, adolescence, rapid growth, or rapid thought processes), they are liable to have epileptic fits. Needless to say, most of the low-threshold people never do have fits but it is this threshold alone that is inherited, and this is the most that families of epileptics should ever feel guilty about. Moreover, it is the most that any epileptic has any right to accuse his family of, in those inevitable bitter moments.

Therefore, if blame had to be apportioned, I had to look for someone else besides my family. If coming from a broken family is a common experience, then a stormy adolescence must surely be, also, at least in Western societies, where old values are continually being undermined and replaced. Moreover, sociologists believe that adolescent traumas are not only inevitable but necessary for the emergence of an independent adult. But higher education does seem to prolong adolescence so that at twenty-one graduates are often still crazy, mixed-up kids rather than the useful members of society which they are expected to exemplify.

Such an extended youth may lead to an inability to accept the adult world and its values. There can be disillusionment, despair and contemplation of, or even attempted suicide. But when the occasional student did actually succeed in killing himself, those of us desperadoes who remained to tell each other the tale were shocked into silencing our moans and complaints, at least for a few weeks.

It was during this teacher training year that my fear of people grew extreme. Facing an ordinary conversation with any of the other students in the Carlton house became quite harrowing. My tiny room was now both haven and prison, a place from which I emerged only with conscious effort. Convinced of being different; frightened that this difference must mean inferiority; lonely, faced with the prospect of a career which was daily becoming more obviously unsuitable, I found life rather burdensome.

I began indulging in something which, on the surface, would appear to be quite innocent, but which I now know to be extremely dangerous for an epileptic. Locked in my room I would spend many hours at a time playing classical music. Prokofiev, Schoenberg, Bloch, Mahler, Grieg — and, inevitably, Chopin. It seemed to have a wonderful effect on me, first of all driving away the blackness, then replacing it with sunshine, and finally bursting into an uncontrollable ecstasy which took hold of me, body, mind and spirit, to float me above the terrors and failures of the day. Music held the answer to everything. Music reconciled all of life into an orderly pattern. It was not a reasonable response but a purely emotional one. And it precipitated T L E in me. More effective than any hard drug, music worked through my whole being to give a glorious 'trip' every time; never a bad one. I would find myself writing on the tiny floor-space with no sense of place or time. I must have written reams of intense, sometimes religious, always ethereal, and mostly incomprehensible rubbish under the influence of music. What a release! But dangerous.

There were other writings as well. Having filled one blue exercise book with angry rejection poetry I managed to fill another with resentment-loneliness-help poetry, nearly all of which contained allusions to my illness, bitterness at the blow God or Nature had dealt me, excuses for my failure with people and general misery. It makes out that I am only half a person — the rest drugs; that all possible struggles have been fought and lost; that all imaginable attempts at learning what I must do to earn people's love and respect have been made and have failed. This blue exercise book fairly screams with terror and pain, cries with grief and loneliness, and entreats someone to come and love this most unlovable person.

Meanwhile, I had managed to convince myself that I was seriously ill and was going to die. I almost wanted it that way because life would otherwise be just too unbearable. Nevertheless, I was terrified of death, especially if it was going to be anything like the death fear which I had experienced so often by then.

It seemed futile even pretending to be whole-hearted and purposeful about the future. I wanted to kill myself, too, but by a most unusual method. The only thought that stopped me carrying it out at first was the absolute conviction that not a soul in the world would be sorry if I died, so it was a pretty hollow sort of revenge.

My method involved the drugs which I absolutely depended upon to cope with the epilepsy. I take enormous quatities of four drugs, including phenobarbitone which would knock out a normal person (someone not used to the drug), in a short while. For some reason we do not crave the drugs as people crave cigarettes, alcohol, even coffee and tea, so there is no help there for us to remember to take them. However, a very real withdrawal is experienced during the changeover from one drug to another — drowsiness, headache, nausea, muscle pain — because our bodies are complaining at the drop in concentration of a certain chemical compound in the blood.

My plan was simply to stop taking the drugs altogether. From what is written in various medical encyclopedias, I gathered that the cessation of anti-convulsant treatment leads to an over-reaction by the body which in turn leads to *status epilepticus.* This is a permanent state of *grand mal.* No sooner does one fit end than another begins, with little or no recovery time in between. By my calculations, it would not take long for me to go into a coma and die. The beauty of it was that I would not have to do anything painful to myself or even perform a conscious act. I had it all worked out.

There was, of course, a quicker way. Beside my bed was a small, brown cupboard in which several huge bottles of pills were kept. The Royal Melbourne Hospital seemed quite willing to give me three months' supply of the stuff. How often did I sit on the floor in front of the old electric fire, with the paper lantern swaying and swaying in the warm air currents, contemplating the contents of that cupboard! I had no idea what could be a lethal dose of any of them, but surely, I reasoned, there would be enough in the cupboard to do the trick. If I made a huge pot of tea and managed to swallow two pills, one big and one little, with each mouthful, I must soon be in a coma.

There were ten students in those two houses which shared a common courtyard. The next two houses were also condemned and also contained students. It was one of them who made me shelve the idea of suicide for ever. She was a Chinese girl, very pretty and petite, but exceedingly lonely. The number of Asians in Melbourne was very small and the white population simply did not know what to say to them. The immigration system meant that children never went to school with someone who was not white;

so although they grew up having learnt of the problems of coloured people in America and Africa, they were inevitably embarrassed and tongue-tied when actually confronted with someone of a different race.

This lass, then, was lonely. She would sometimes speak to me, as we stood at our respective front gates, of how she enjoyed walking on moonlight nights in the big, old cemetery across the way, and of how peaceful it was there, how the dead had no problems. I thought it strange — but thought no more. One day I heard on the radio that a Chinese girl had gone to the law cloisters at 3 a.m., poured kerosene over herself and set it alight. She had run, screaming with agony, around the old cloisters for nearly an hour until she mercifully died before anyone could bring so much as a shirt to help put out the flames. I just knew it must be Jan. A tremendous fuss was made in the Melbourne papers over the plight of overseas students and the front pages showed photographs of Jan's windowless cupboard room, furnished only with a mattress, a cupboard and a fruit box, on which was a milk bottle with a single daffodil in it. Nobody had known — but nobody had asked. For me, the shock was appalling. I decided to go on living.

It was just crazy for me to contemplate teaching. Frankly, I didn't really contemplate it much at all. This teacher training was just the next stage. Our course was largely theory with a total of nine weeks of teaching practice. I was endeavouring to teach General Science to the middle school bracket — trying to ignore the fact that, except in Biology, my scientific knowledge went up to and stopped at Newton. The first teaching practice session was moderately terrible; the second was a foreshortened disaster and the third, a blot on my memory. I failed teaching practice. However, as I passed all other subjects and science teachers were in demand, I was pushed through with a strictly supervised supplementary examination.

By no means everybody is custom-built for teaching. It

takes a strong personality, a one-track mind, a good sense of humour and a certain amount of acting — but above all, self-confidence. There is no shame in being unable to control an unwilling class of forty screaming thirteen-year-olds of very mixed abilities. But I walked obstinately straight into the middle of every practice session, naively believing that this time, the class would act just as I was fondly convinced I used to behave during school.

There was one counterbalance to the desolation I felt. The big event in my week was the University Choral Society meeting, every Monday. It had about two hundred members and was of a high standard. I went on an Inter-Varsity Choral Festival in Adelaide, Australia's city for the arts, where about a thousand students gathered and sang and got drunk and did all the things that students will.

I had never touched alcohol until third year in college. From somewhere I had heard that drinking was not a good idea for epileptics so, feeling like a martyr, I refrained. (Actually, I had once attempted to drink half a glass of Melbourne Bitter, but to my sweet tooth it tasted foul.) At special dinners in college, people liked to have me on their table as it meant more wine per head! Therefore, when I did start drinking, my susceptibility was very high. Even now, two glasses of wine and I am floating in the land of multi-coloured sugar crystals. Fortunately, I just do not enjoy it very much. I say fortunately because there are many reasons why epileptics should try to be teetotallers if they can.

Alcohol increases the possibility of *grand mal*, acting like a poison in combination with the normal drugs. Also, the effects of alcohol can be doubled because of the drugs. Apart from that, too many late nights are likely to precipitate an attack, and once an epileptic has good drug control, he will appreciate his freedom from attacks so much that his resistance to such invitations will be sure to grow. Alcohol damages the brain tissue in normal people — so how much more may it not damage an epileptic? We take enough drugs without asking our bodies to cope with an even worse mixture. But alcohol is such an integral part of life for so many people that pub time can be an unendurable reminder of an epileptic's singularity. So a compromise might be necessary — have a glass (preferably shandy); make it last; and don't ask for another! It is honestly not worth all the extra reactions we will probably get.

But here my defiance won over common sense. So, on the last evening of the festival, when everyone was having a good time at a party I was sitting in the hall (on the floor) of somebody's house in Adelaide, utterly intoxicated after only four glasses of rather bad red wine. Someone was sitting beside me in a similar state and we had a long discussion in each other's arms. This was the beginning of a beautiful friendship — mainly developed through the mail; because Chris was from the Taswegian contingent. We had something extra in common. Chris also had a grand secret. His brother was autistic and had neither spoken nor communicated with people in twenty-three years, although he had invented what amounted to the binary system of numbers, and had knitted an enormous rug with an elaborate pattern of his own design without a single mistake, starting from one corner. Once I began to talk to Chris I ceased to be frightened of him as a male but rather became interested in him as a person. A small crack had appeared in my impenetrable, adolescent-epileptic armour.

The festival began with a fortnight's stay in Quorn, a gold-rush ghost town near the Red Centre. You can tell how prosperous a township once was by the number of abandoned pubs. Quorn had been very rich — we were billeted in all the pubs. There I had an interesting meeting with a real poet who lived in one of the many derelict houses. Then we all crowded into coaches and went back to Adelaide where we performed 'The Choir Invisible' by Joubert. But it was not we who were invisible — it was the audience.

Then my former life of lectures and loneliness was resumed, with an occasional letter from Chris. He was a keen mountaineer, as well as a good singer, and he would write from all over the snow-covered alps of Tasmania. Sometimes the letter would have become very wet from the snow dripping off Chris as he thawed from his latest twenty-mile walk.

The biggest shock of my entire life up till then came during this year. All the Dip Ed. students were put through a rigorous, three-hour intelligence test as a prelude to our lectures on the subject. I had taken similar tests at school a few times and one teacher had disclosed that my I Q was higher than hers. Fortunately I did not know what I Q meant, so it did no immediate harm. Now, an I Q rating means nothing in relation to one's success in life in any field whatsoever, but it is somehow very disturbing to know one's own rating. After an extensive lecture on the subject we were each given our score in a sealed envelope. Mine was 155, which means M E N S A – genius. As far as I know, there was only one other Dip. Ed. student that year with a M E N S A rating. This was a real and sudden shock, and I cried for weeks about it, saying to Chopin in my little room, 'It's not fair. It's not fair. What chance have I got with a rating like that?' I still believe that unless people with such a rating have enough sense not to let it set them apart from other people, it can only be a handicap for them.

My only consolation was that in real terms, the epilepsy took me down at least twenty or thirty points, besides, I was so stunned that the subsequent lectures dealing with all the other factors that affect the final I Q rating, were virtually lost on me. But upbringing, education, family background, illness, determination, single-mindedness, ambition, perseverance, ability to be side-tracked – a thousand associated factors put me right back to being a very ordinary student.

The Wind had done his utmost. My coat was close around me. Now the Sun was going to try. Apart from Chris's warm feelings, I found a brief saviour in Dr C., an apparently mild, obscure and gentle character who occasionally lectured to us on psychology. I went to him in dismay with my I Q rating in its tear-stained, grubby envelope, and poured out all my fears and troubles to him. He was a good listener. He decided to try a Rauschach (Blot) Test on me, as an experiment, but his real aim was to convince me that I was a normal adolescent with fairly normal problems. The blots and smudges were very confusing. Some of the patterns meant nothing to me at all. In others I related to the colours, but not the shapes. How he could judge anything of my personality from that, I still have no idea. This man was gentle and patient, coaxing answers from me but not forcing them. I had to wait a week for his verdict. It certainly gave me something to think about.

Dr. C. was not quite sure why I was trying to be a teacher, either. But he did say a few very wise things. Firstly, that my views of the opposite sex were a bit underdeveloped but would blossom in their own time. Secondly, that either I would become a first-class teacher or else be a complete failure. (That was honest). Then, if I was the sort of person who failed at teaching, I would find something, by twenty-four or twenty-five years of age, that I would do extremely well. So — if teaching was not the right thing (I had already lived through two three-week practice sessions by that time), I was not to worry too much. I would find my slot in society eventually. Three years later I returned to Dr C. to tell him that his prophecy had come true.

9

That fourth year at university was also the year of my twenty-first birthday. This, which is a great event in many people's lives, was a source of dread for me. My elder brother had just married, after great arguments and bitter tears as to which parent should attend the wedding, if neither would submit to being under the same roof as the other. I did not want a similar argument over any celebration that I might have, which is where my widely travelled, broad-minded, stimulating aunt and uncle stepped in. They gave a small dinner at their home, which we followed by seeing the film *Funny Girl*. *Funny Girl* was a revelation for me, because Barbra Streisand is such an individual and does what suits her, which the rest of the world can like or go hang. People either love her or hate her almost immediately. She does not compromise her personality by trying to be what almost everybody may like. She just is — herself. Sweet inspiration!

It began to dawn on me that it could be an interesting experiment *not* to care what people think. I had spent my life letting my real self sleep, trying to be like other people, trying desperately to be what I thought people wanted me to be. I had never discovered who I really was or what I was like. The fear of how awful I must look while in the throes of a fit had carried through to every waking minute. Soon I found a new theme song to put as a challenge alongside that verse from *Old Coat*. It was Streisand singing:

> *Nobody can tell you*
> *There's only one song worth singing —*
> *Don't let them compel you*
> *Because it cuts them up to see someone like you!*

You've got to — make your own kind of music,
Sing you own special song —
Make your own kind of music,
Even if nobody else sings along.

So, perhaps I might have something worthwhile to offer, after all. Streisand implies that everyone does, that everyone *must* be himself, first. It was towards the end of that year, despite my abysmal failure in the classroom and with *Funny Girl* in mind, that I started walking around town looking at my feet and shoulders and anything else I could see. A feeling of selfness was finally dawning. I would grin and say, 'Hey — this is me. This is me walking through Carlton. I'm a person. A real, live person!' At twenty-one, I had just discovered identity.

At last, I was beginning to fight back, and positively. Maybe here was the beginning of the unsteady, fluttering progress, of fits and new starts, which might eventually lift me out of all this darkness and into the warm sunshine. Next year would certainly be freedom, of a kind. I would have to become somebody and something if I was to survive. Looking at myself from the new viewpoint that identity had given, I decided that it would be quite a challenge — and very hard work. I was to become an adult epileptic in the normal adult world. The testing point was just the other side of Christmas.

There had been a great exodus of Australian teachers to Canada, where the pay and conditions were reputedly better. This left a big hole in the pool of local, experienced teachers. However, desperate as they were, it soon became evident that the Victorian Education Department was not eager to take on people like me. Handicapped teachers, so I was told, were paid on an hourly basis. There was no provision for advancement up the public service scale and contracts could be terminated without notice. But I did not feel handicapped; all my bad fits were coming in the evenings and tension did not seem to make any difference. I am much more likely to react when the tension has gone, in the same way that I get a 'Sunday headache', once the week's excitement is behind me. Australia is not kind to anybody whom they consider to be handicapped. As a nation it is too healthy. If I was trying to emigrate back to my country, I would not be allowed in! Epilepsy is one of the 'proscribed diseases' which specifically prevents application for emigration to Australia. So although I felt, and looked, perfectly healthy, I might as well have gone into the interview stark naked, painted blue with a ring through my nose, my hair shaved off, smoking a cheroot and in the last stage of *delirium tremens*. The effect would have been the same.

Being too proud to submit myself to all the department's humiliations and provisos, I decided to look for a job outside the state system. Also, it was becoming obvious that my mother and I had vastly different ideas as to what I could and couldn't do. My strong reaction against her picture of me living quietly at home, doing some obscure, back-bench job in the Ministry (a perfectly reasonable ambition for someone like me), was probably a great help in counteracting my low self-esteem. I was determined to do something; unfortunately my motives came from pure recalcitrance, not the more estimable independence. I decided that I must cut the umbilical cord and go right away, to another state.

But it was not so simple — just to leave. We had a comfortable and convenient surburban home, cream brick, triple-fronted and built sufficiently far off the ground to let a few cool currents go under the floorboards in summer. There were two huge, flowering gum trees in the front garden, one red and one pink, which were full of bees in the spring. The rest of the garden was overcrowded with presents I had given my mother — luculia, roses, camellias, flowering cherry; plants were a nice sort of gift because I was really giving them to myself as well.

Before I had always been within phoning distance of

home. But perhaps that had been the trouble. Perhaps I needed a testing-ground which would provide true independence. Fits I could handle, couldn't I? It would not be much of a wrench to leave anybody behind. I was certain that this new start (and how many of those had I tried up until then?) would make everything better.

Having relatives in Sydney, 600 miles away, I travelled north and was gladly taken in as a junior science teacher by a day-girl convent which had quite a few lay teachers. I did not tell them of my epilepsy — I was still smarting from the humiliating interviews with the Victorian Education Department.

Sydney is certainly a beautiful place, although as a staunch Melbournite, I am loathe to admit it. The climate is that much warmer than Melbourne, but not tropical as in Brisbane, a further 600 miles north again. People grow rubber plants, date palms and banana shoots in their front gardens. They have hedges made of shrimp plants and there are public baths every few miles. And the surf beaches . . . . My new convent was within a few miles of one of them so I was able to indulge my great love of body-surfing every day after school for a whole term. It was unusually hot and there was a severe drought. In five months there was not a cloud in the sky, let alone a drop of rain. The cicadas thought it was still Christmas in May! I revelled in the warmth of the ever-rolling ocean.

My need to fight against all the physical limitations of epilepsy continued. Being a fairly strong swimmer, I knew that I could always win against the sea, which doubled the excitement I usually get from those glorious waves. There was never any doubt in my mind that I would come out as safely as I went in — and that was the last thing I could say about the classroom. Surfing was a great opportunity to get rid of all the anger and frustrations of teaching.

When I had a hard day, or when something bad happened to me, I really thought that I was the only person in the world burdened by a terrible combination of experiences, and I felt thoroughly persecuted. It did not occur to me, all through that time, that a similar fear or failure might have been experienced by ninety per cent of the rest of the population as well. I had not yet discovered *Desiderata* which simply says 'Be yourself . . . .' But I should have remembered old Polonius' advice: '. . . Above all things, to thine own self be true . . . .' The pupils at the convent probably sensed that I was not being myself. Children are quick to notice the chink in the armour of an adult, and they played up to my every wrong move. The last straw was when I discovered a lot of girls cheating in tests, having been to mass confession only the previous day. I had assumed their honesty as well as their attention, because of my own interest in lessons. But it was a shaky assumption to build on. Many a time I had been the ringleader in a teacher-baiting session. How convenient it was to forget the way we had also picked certain teachers to pieces!

One of the worst characteristics a teacher can have is indecision. In any situation the children must know where they stand with authority, so that whether the action is just or not, it must be consistent and swift. Being so unsure of myself in this, my first professional position, I hesitated when I saw any of the girls misbehaving. I wanted to be fair to them and not punish the wrong ones, or be too severe when it was not warranted. Another reason for my hesitation was often a minor seizure, possibly brought on by the rapidity of events leading up to the misconduct. The three or four minutes following an attack would give the girls time to argue, cajole and generally break up the continuity of a lesson, without me being able to answer.

Once, in despair over one of these frequent interruptions, I became so incensed that I thumped a particularly defiant little twelve-year old on the back. She showed no emotion and I thumped her again and again, trying to get her to react in some way. This incident showed me what could happen if I tried to contain the anger for too long. It was not a pretty scene. Could such a sudden storm be attributed to epilepsy? The thought frightened me into allowing the children to trample all over me for the rest of the term.

This is not to say that all or most epileptics may find themselves having either *petit mal* or uncontrolled rages in front of a class. But before deciding to teach, just ask yourself honestly whether straight questions, when you are tired or confused, sometimes cause a slight seizure. If they do, then you still may be an excellent teacher, especially if you can make up for these attacks by your methods, extensive knowledge and intelligent handling of the children. Perhaps this careful self-examination could apply to all prospective teachers, whether epileptic or not. I would have had to give myself nought out of ten for all three qualities. Children just won't tolerate indecision, whatever the cause.

Occasionally I would experience a full-length T L E during an afternoon and the children took advantage of my obvious confusion, as children will. It was not fair on them to expect anything else. I never once cried, not in front of the class, anyway, but I gave up trying to do anything but baby sit, about half-way through the term.

In short, I was a hopeless teacher: easily side-tracked by some cunning little girls who enjoyed putting irrelevant questions; unable to put down disturbances by a look or a caustic word but, rather, finding it necessary to harangue a class with long lectures on behaviour; appalled at the huge amount of preparation and marking which seemed necessary; having nobody to let off steam to after school; I must have looked like a caged lion, striding helplessly up and down, making growling noises. The onlookers are quite unafraid of such a beast, and will often tease and provoke it. I have no happy memories of that frightful term. A teacher must have a thick skin; I took every childish taunt personally, so that my idea of what those ordinary little girls thought of me grew to ridiculous proportions.

Unhappily, my living arrangements were also bleak.

I had bed and board in the home of one of the convent girls. Her mother's idea of board was a bowl of cornflakes (always unaccountably stale) in the morning, a heated-up pie and half a can of beans in the evening, all accompanied by unlimited cups of weak tea. This was insufficient to prepare any teacher for today's or tomorrow's gruelling tasks. I was soon lonely and unhappy to the point of shock, quite apart from the traumas at school. Evidently, the new start had not come off.

There was one good experience that came out of this terrible three months. I started going to see the famous Sydney production of *Hair*, the 'tribal, love-rock, musical', and soon became a *Hair* addict, going in to King's Cross to see a performance every Saturday for nine weeks. How a prim, unworldly, quietly raised, inexperienced lass like me even got to find out about it, I cannot remember. Sydney's flower people — the hippies around Paddington — were much further advanced than anything to be found in Melbourne. I would sit in the blazing sun outside the theatre and watch everything, greedily taking in the attitudes and imagined lives of the milling crowds. They dressed in weird clothes, they wore flowers and bare feet, headbands, long skirts, jeans held together by a few threads. They leaned out of windows in twos and threes, made love on the lawns. Here were possibilities for an unheard-of freedom of spirit that life so far had not taught me. I did not belong to them — yet. But I felt comfortable and at peace, just watching them, being there. Here were people who did not care about collecting things around them, who had apparently strong relationships with lots of other people. They believed such relationships, such caring, were infinitely more important than things.

None of the flower people was an island. They belonged to something real and apparently good, they said and did what came naturally. I have since discovered that this intensely strong peace movement was based on heroin-pushing and petty in-fighting. The power of their words had gone to the heads of the original leaders, and they were no longer the simple human beings that they tried to pretend they were. This became especially true of New York. But, whatever the true story behind *Hair* and the people involved in it, and even the hippies, the lasting impression on me was one of peace, love, freedom and happiness. What it said to me was, if you don't like what you are doing then for goodness sake — stop! Don't try to be like other people. Being yourself is sufficient. I learned the music of the show by heart, bought the record and danced as crazily as a dervish in my own room. It was a drug, a pair of rose-coloured glasses, a new hope — a last hope, as I thought.

Thus I began to relaxing my careful watch on how I looked to other people, how plain I was and how uninteresting. *Hair* told me that everybody has got something worthwhile — everybody — just as Streisand had urged me to sing my own special song. With a tremendous effort of will-power I started the search for anything in me worth salvaging from the mess.

It is not so strange that, having cut myself off from people, I turned to other things for clues to a new view of life. *Funny Girl* and the incomparable Streisand; *Hair* with its great variety of people all embraced by the tribe; *Godspell* and its simplicty of thought and action which denied the charms of sophistication; the novels of Patrick White, with their wonderful portraits of lone eccentrics who actually prefer few or no real friends to a million nodding acquaintances.

I was not quite ready to stick two fingers in the air at what people thought. But the process had begun, and *Hair* helped. It was a tremendous revelation to see someone dancing around the stage in very little except for a headband, defying anybody to question what he had: 'I got life, brother; I got laughs, sister; I got freedom, mother; I got good times, man; I got crazy ways, daughter; I got million-dollar charm, cousin; I got headaches and toothaches and bed times too like you . . . I got my hair, I got my head . . . eyes . . . brains . . . ears . . . .' When it was all counted up he had quite a lot really, enough to be going on with — and it finally occured to me that so did I. Unfortunately, there was no miraculous change in my woeful lack of ability as a teacher. Trying to practise all that peace-love-freedom theory was very difficult, especially as I was alone, with no one to reinforce my frail convictions. Ideas bumped about inside my head, resolutions, plans — If you don't like what you are doing, for goodness sake, stop! They were right. But how to make such a decision? Finally it was made for me. I became involved in a cruelty case, in which the Mother Superior beat a child all over her body because I had casually remarked that the child was a ringleader and I could do nothing with her. My inability to control my students was my fault, but I felt obligated to support the Mother Superior's action. I think she was rather relieved when I gave notice. I was stunned, having failed horribly in my first real job. Self-respect was at an all time low. The wobbly writings in my blue exercise book from this time are almost illegible. I left Sydney with an awful sense of failure, having shelved the possibility suggested by *Hair* and *Funny Girl* for the moment, and with a ready finger wagging at my blanket excuse for all my failures.

10

The next scene was enacted back in the Nest. When I returned home, my mother suggested that I was not cut out for teaching, and that I should try something else. Of course, she was right, but my limited information about careers left me unenthusiastic about any of the alternatives. What could I do? Trained for teaching, but terrified to try another school, believing myself to be banned from almost every interesting profession, yet wanting to join and succeed in a profession, I had no idea where to start next.

Thoroughly demoralized, I was also thoroughly out of pocket. My mother was not wealthy, and the family weren't likely to help unless I was in absolute dire straits, or getting married. I was neither, so I scanned local newspapers for a job — any job — just to tide me over until the one and only job came along. Someone was advertising for a 'quick, alert, young person' to train in a middle-management type job, in a factory. When I got to the interview I was deemed unsuitable for the work advertised, but they offered me another job, actually working on the factory assembly line.

This employment was preceded by the usual wrangle over my epilepsy. I was taken on as a temporary. It is obviously dangerous for even the most controlled epileptic to work with heavy machinery. Even if we are only having one *grand mal* per year there is a good chance that we will have it while bending over some whirring machinery. It only has to happen once.

There is a less obvious danger, just as great as the possibility of a *grand mal*, if you really decided that what you most want to do is create super-accurate screw threads, or be part of an assembly plant and watch machines grow before your very eyes. This is that the continual hum of loud machinery, the sparks of cutting tools and flames of welding torches, along with the piped music that so many factories have now, combine to make the possibility of frequent T L E attacks very great. The management might never find out — but who wants to spend half of their working day wrestling with the Terror? Another elementary consideration is that the inevitable night shifts and overtime completely ruin one's sleep patterns — one of the most vital things to maintain, along with regular meals and drugs, in the fight to stave off *grand mal*.

Although my new job was only in light industry, I spent several afternoons fighting my little devil. The work I turned out was automatic, but of extra-low standard. I lasted three weeks.

It was not the early start that put me off; nor was it the all too brief half-hour lunch; nor was it really the soggy egg sandwiches and weak tea served up in a lunch room with no windows. It was not even the monotony of the job, which was its outstanding quality. Every so often, somebody gave me a large box of long metal things which looked like nails without ends. I had to dip them in flux, which smelt nauseating, and to squash them, one by one, between the jaws of an electric heat-squashing machine. Then somebody else came and took the results away and told me to work faster — I was too slow and deliberate; I did not have 'the knack'. Pick up, dip, hold in place, squash, lift, clonk, ad infinitum. How can anyone do this sort of job for long? It must be easier if you just look upon it as a way of earning money. Perhaps I might have graduated to trotting around and distributing the boxes after five years or so.

What made me most upset was that nobody told me what these little metal things were used for. The best I can do is to imagine they were the ends of screwdrivers, before they are given a plastic handle. But I hate to think they might have been bullets, or rivets, or bicycle spokes, or saucepan handles or the ends of electric beaters or some gadget that no person can do without — well, anything, in fact, without me knowing it.

For want of something better to do, I decided to return to the Education Department and put my case once more. Several people advised me to ask for a non-teaching post. So I was interviewed, examined and even stripped naked by the medical officer — goodness only knows why. The solution they came up with was a provisional but positive one. Since I was medically unfit to teach they would do me the honour of taking me on as a non-combatant and even give me a job. To my utter amazement the department was actually interested in my degree! That strange mixture of scientific history, French, logic, English and biology seemed highly promising to them. I would be useful as a course designer for the middle years at school.

So, with renewed interest, I started work again. The office was in a huge, white building with small, square windows, but our particular area had no windows at all. Being addicted to sunshine I always find this frustrating. More importantly, the exaggerated whiteness of neon lights, the buzzing in them when a 'starter' is faulty, the flashing of the older bulbs — all this is anathema to the epileptic. The lack of fresh air and the controlled atmosphere are no help either. The result? Just as many afternoons spent in the company of my devil as when I worked in the factory. By that time I was learning what sort of things would precipitate T L E — but there was very little I could do about working in this office.

The job at least sounded hopeful. Well, I had my own partitioned office, telephone, chair, visitor's chair, papers, pens and even a small laboratory; in fact only one thing was lacking — work. The four men in the office seemed very surprised when I asked what I was supposed to be doing. Why — nothing, of course! I got tired of reading novels and drawing patterns on the paper. The men had a huge graph on which they drew up the continuing, daily progress of the Stock Exchange. Some read newspapers and did the cryptic crossword; some rang up their wives. One even marked papers for an obscure technical subject. We had a general meeting with the science course administrator every Thursday. We were a committee, so we discussed things in the usual manner of committees everywhere — for instance, how long we were going to discuss things for, what things we were going to discuss, what things we would put off discussing until next week, what we had discussed last week and who was going to report on this week's meeting. By then it was time to go home. I would look around at these men pretending to be so earnest and solemn and I could often do nothing but laugh — except when it was really too pathetic for mirth. I wrote a rude poem about committees once and circulated it during a meeting to prevent me from having the screaming abdabs at all this balderdash. They took it seriously and several of them worried over that poem for some time.

So much for being a highly paid non-combatant. I believe it is immoral to take money for doing nothing, so I wrote a course in the History and Philosophy of Science for second-year level — in my spare time, naturally. I got permission to have it trialled in two safe private schools. Nobody even patted me on the head for my efforts. I was fed up with playing gin rummy for two hours every lunchtime, so I finally stomped up to the Head and told him what I thought of his easy money establishment. I told him the truth about what went on, every day, in our office. He went white with fury. I was hounded, flouted, cross-examined, intimidated, treated like a guilty scullery-maid and finally given the sack by this crinkle-curled man, this supposedly friendly boss who invited everyone to come to him at any time — his door was always open — and he would see what he could do. He told me that if I wanted to work I could go back to real teaching and good luck to me. He was half out of his chair and purple before he had finished. On his recommendation I was given a place in the largest high school in Victoria. A clever move, on his part.

This little scene was indicative of a change. Perhaps at

least the painful, ingrown toenail effect of the last eight years was diminishing. The final pages of the oh-so-blue exercise book show a different trend; they even change colour. Sometimes they are pink with the excitement of discovery! 'The beautiful sunshine is coming back into my life . . . I am becoming happy . . .' it reads — and that is before the awful interview! Sometimes pale green with fresh thoughts; bright red with righteous anger; in places, even golden with hope and white with pure relief. And sometimes blue — of course.

11

It was with many misgivings that I went back to teaching proper. The department had all the files on my medical record and I was the lowest of the low. Paid by the hour, unable to protest, no long-term agreement and no superannuation — I was going to be a dogsbody.

In Great Britain, anyone with a history of epilepsy, however well-controlled, would not even be considered for teaching. In Australia, the Education Departments made sure that they reserved the right to throw me out at a moment's notice — which is not much better. With very little effort, and some grounds, I could have let myself believe that I was a second-class — no, third class — citizen (in Australia, women were still second-class in a number of ways). The superannuation issue was a real thorn in my side. The money one gets on retiring from a job can be almost equivalent to the last salary earned; much better than going on a state pension. Most professionals in all fields had this sort of insurance — but it was subject to a medical test. Epilepsy was one of the 'diseases' which universally prevented anyone from receiving superannuation. Being so young, that did not worry me much, but the basic inequality of it did. Surely I was a good risk if they thought I was going to die before being eligible for any payments? They might have done a bit of checking up of their facts with someone like Dr Ebeling. If I did die, they would have all my money to throw around on somebody else. But the insurance firms did not look at things that way.

As well as being excluded from a whole range of professions, I can't get life assurance, company retirment benefit and many other things including a mortgage — all because of my E E G reading. What do all those official bodies expect me to do? Subside into a hole and submit to it all with bowed head? No wonder I went down fighting like a cat every time.

At least I was back to teaching, back to my interminable chain of new starts. At this school the classes were enormous (average, forty) and yet we were expected to take them single-handed for double practical lessons and, what was often worse, double theory lessons. Fortunately, at my school we were never given a double lesson in the timetable until fourth year, but if we had been, I think my reaction would have been no much better than the reaction of this lot. Chaotic. Impossible, unnerving, tragic — and a plain waste of everybody's time. Even worse, there was no laboratory assistant, so after a simple lesson involving test tubes, Bunsen burners and twelve-year olds I was left alone to deal with the sad remains.

It seemed that these children's greatest joy in life was destruction. I would jump down one child's throat for experimenting with the relative combustion of wooden and plastic rulers, only to find that another child was trying a similar experiment on the hair of the girls in front. This patched up, I would smell burning rubber and on the way to its source would have to stop a water fight while also trying to find the chief participants in a chalk fight. There was rarely one piece of undamaged apparatus to be found after such a session. The children were evidently bored. But the saddest thing of all were the three or four children who were obviously keen on science and tried desperately to catch my attention for explanations or answers, without success. My first priority had to be the attempted control of those who didn't care two sticks for science lessons. It soon became clear that I was a genuine disaster as a high school science teacher.

But it could not be all due to epilepsy. I had no real fear of having a fit in front of a class. *Grand mals* came only after the relaxation of tension — I knew that by now —

and lessons were all tension! Minor fits, especially T L E, were a problem, though — a big problem.

It cannot help one's esteem in the eyes of a normal, energetic, mixed class if one goes blank for several minutes at least once in every lesson, and nearly always after being asked a question. This happened to me too often to think about. I would be in the middle of an explanation of, say, acceleration, when I would falter and stop, only to recover as if I did not have a clue what I was trying to teach. The lump of misery, the dreadful desire to scream would nearly break the surface of my throat, but there was no choice. I had to take myself right back to the beginning and go through once again. Admittedly, I was unsure of the material — only one jump ahead of the children, in fact, with some of the work. With some classes I was plain scared and it took real will-power even to set foot in the door of their room, expecially if I was having a succession of *petit mals* dreading the onset of T L E in front of them.

It is my personal experience that a great percentage of all types of seizures can be controlled from within. Using plenty of mind energy to promote will-power, an attack may be curbed before it takes hold. The opposite is also true. In a set of shaky circumstances, just let yourself panic and you are likely to get what you ask for.

So it was that, letting myself go too often, T L E took hold more than necessary and all my laborious preparations for each class went right down the drain. Children are not patient, and many of my fourteen-year olds were quite bright. They wrote me off fairly early as an unstimulating, boring, crabby old idiot. (I was twenty-two). They had a nickname for me which they called me to my face: Miss Chook. As I walked down the corridors I was always followed by a lot of loud clucking and cackling. I pretended not to notice, but oh — it must have shown on my face! I was desperately unhappy — again.

Just before Easter, the episode of the paté occurred. I was

still living at home with my mother who, as usual, was doing everything. I was allowed to dry the dishes, but little else. As a child I was never given the chance to learn cooking, which frustrated me because I really wanted to be creative in this small way.

One night I brought home a pound of chicken livers. Someone had given me a recipe for chicken liver paté which seemed simple enough, and I was looking forward to making it. Mum, a good plain cook, who never tried anything new, found the splodgy soft, little bundle and threw it in the rubbish bin. That did it. I exploded. She never heard the end of all her suppression, oppression, depression (and all the rest of it) of me. I found a flat that weekend and moved in, refusing even to give her my address.

These occasional outbursts of temper were beginning to worry me. Not that I felt I was in the wrong, but somehow it seemed so different from my normal self. It had happened before when I had thumped the little convent girl and also when I had told the general administrator of the non-combatant teacher's division what I thought of his holiday camp. Now I had seen red with my mother. It was not the first time. I decided it was worth asking my new specialist's opinion. Since returning from Sydney I had been with a new neurologist, back in Collins Street. My long struggle with Dr Ebeling was finally over. We both knew that he had won. The new man was pleasant, almost bald, with square rimless glasses. He did at least listen. Was such violence so abnormal in a character who was usually the epitome of mildness? Or perhaps it was just a safety valve which occasionally erupted in a stressful situation instead of the alternative of a T L E attack?

Unfortunately I made the mistake of putting diagnoses in the doctors' mouth, which they often don't counteract. I was dismayed with what this neurologist came up with — valium. The brown tube, filled with small yellow pills, remained untouched for many months. For me, the word valium had associations with nervous breakdowns and other drastic conditions. Actually valium is often used for severe epilepsy, and when a patient has gone into the state of *status epilepticus,* valium is injected directly into the veins. Valium is also given, frequently, as an addition to anti-convulsant drugs, when there is undue distress. Eventually I came to accept it and allowed myself to be prescribed a tiny amount daily. I think it does prevent me from being too unreasonable, too often.

But if it was natural for me to act like that, should not the fury be allowed to take its course, rather than be buried under pacifying compounds? I still don't know. During these moments of righteous indignation, something takes over my brain (perhaps it is my own little devil?) and, using all the word-power at its disposal, continues to rave until I realize what is happening, at which stage it swiftly dried up. But it usually has had time to make the point effectively. Frankly, I wish I could do it more often; I might get more done to my own satisfaction! It is wonderful to blast one's own absolute truth at some offender and see him reduced to a heap of astonished jelly. It clears the air and makes me look forward to dinner.

And so, as a result of one such flare-up, I found myself renting a flat. Although it had never occurred to me, I now know that it is rather hazardous for an epileptic to take a flat alone. But here my natural rebelliousness was victorious. The necessity of having people around, 'just in case', served only to remind me of my disability, to prevent me from thinking clearly, and to make me chafe against this bit of unfairness. Having such a degree of real independence was marvellous for the morale — there was nobody to check up on me. I was responsible only to myself.

My new flat had a large bed-sitting-room, a large, light kitchen with bathroom partition, and a shared toilet and laundry facilities. It had an enormous garden, both back and front, like most Australian suburban houses, and since nobody in the other two flats was interested, I became the proud owner of twenty-one rose bushes and a potato patch. The kitchen and a little gas stove, all of one cubic foot, not counting the lift-up side ring. To an accomplished cook this contraption might have seemed a bit constricting, but to an aspiring one it simply glowed with possibilities. I got myself a few cookery-books and rapidly learnt the joys of everything — from fried bread to roast chicken — that could just fit in the cubic foot oven. My *piece de resistance* was baked stuffed aubergine.

Fortunately for me, the stove was set in an old fireplace area, with a low mantelpiece, so it would have been difficult to be harmed by having a *grand mal* in front of it. The best thing for we epileptic cooks to do is to train ourselves to cook on the back rings and turn the handles to the wall, so that we soon do it without thinking. There are myriad small bits of common sense that can make it possible for a fairly well controlled epileptic to live alone. A bit of thought and planning for safety is all that one needs to open up the great prospect of true independence. The hot water system can be regulated so that it is never hot enough to scald us if we should have a *grand mal* in the shower and turn the cold tap off as we fall. If the electric, gas or open fires are made safe enough for a toddler, then that is a good indication that they are safe enough for us. I had to find all these things out the hard way . . . . I wish now that I had 'faced reality' and applied some common sense to my own position. But serious *grand mals* were only occuring every two or three months by that time and I anticipated no danger. The worst was yet to come.

My spirits soared. I bought curtains, rugs and cushions, tables and bookcases. This place was really mine! Personal achievements, however insignificant they may seem, are terribly important to an epileptic. It is all part of the pressing need for independence. With independence comes confidence and with confidence comes ability, pride and usefulness. It all snowballs into a renewal of a reason for living.

Not having the family continually hovering over my 'health' (that is for people of ninety-plus in bath chairs!), I slowly began to see through the thick fog which had encompassed me for so long. I began to look objectively at the direction life was taking; to realize that I dreaded every school day, that I sighed over every careless workbook, that I was disillusioned by the number of children who did not care two hoots if they got nought for a science test, that I was bone weary.

There were forty periods in a week and I taught for thirty-two of them, as well as filling in for absent teachers during another three or four lessons. It meant that I had twenty-four consecutive science lessons to teach, which gave me no breather from Monday lunch-time until Thursday recess. No wonder I dragged myself into each lesson looking low-spirited; no wonder the children got the better of me by half-way through it. The odds were desperately unfair. I was not alone either. At the end of first term, twenty per cent of the teaching staff gave notice.

About this time I made a new friend. Our dear, old brown-eyed, black-haired, smooth-coated dog had died from cancer. Like most dogs she had been a great friend – the sort who is never horrified at anything you might say, but listens patiently, looking at you with loving eyes. I had never known any cats very well and did not like them by comparison. But there are always exceptions – and I met her. She used to live in the house before it was made into flats, and her owners had taken her to their new home, fifteen miles away. One day I saw a thin, slinky, coal-black cat with wild eyes, lurking near the potato patch. She obviously thought that she belonged here. After travelling over six months to find her former home, she was now quite wild, having fought for her food all the way. It took me weeks before I could coax her into the kitchen, and months before she would allow herself to be stroked. But she had definitely adopted me and it was she who became my friend. She was a beautiful cat, once she started eating properly: slim with a fine, small head like a Siamese; I called her Sloopy. She followed me everywhere and watched me with her glinting, impatient eyes.

As I sat on the back steps in the morning sun, drinking tea, or sat under the trees in the evening watching the glorious sunsets which set fire to the sky in Australia, I would talk to Sloopy and ask her opinion. Somehow animals are so much more receptive than people. They have all the time in the world to listen and are less likely to interrupt your chain of thought. Also, and more importantly, you are much more likely to tell them the truth. That is one way of finding it out for yourself.

With Sloopy's aid I realized that I could scarcely digest breakfast for fear of the day ahead, or eat supper for fear of the consequences of the day behind. I resolved to think very carefully, not of what I ought to be doing, or of what might please other people, but of what in the whole world I would prefer to do, rather than face another term of those screaming kids. The answer came loud and clear — I wanted to work in a bookshop. The things that made me most content were music, gardening and books. The first two were hobbies — unlikely professions. But books — there was a world in itself, a means of learning to enjoy the whole of life, including the working part.

The idea grew and blossomed. I would sit in the classroom on hot, drowsy afternoons, half-listening to the buzz of children talking, the rest of me (in spirit) surrounded by shelves of crisp new novels with bright covers. There was no hope of discussing the idea with friends or family. Being a shop assistant simply did not come into any of their spheres of experience — or taste. So, after an earnest discussion with Sloopy and a particularly rough week at school, I just gave notice and walked out, light-headed maybe, but light-hearted too.

12

And what is so dreadful about working in a shop? In a professional and landed family like mine, trade was not thought exactly nice; tradesmen were considered necessary evils. But the great attraction about such a job for me was the total absence of professional dictates on health standards, and all the complications and debarments from accrued benefits. I no longer wanted to slave my days away in utter misery all for the sake of professional status, security and salary.

So I marched into the biggest bookshop in the city of Melbourne and asked to see the manager. He was in, surprisingly, and he saw me. In ten minutes I had a job as a shop assistant starting Monday. No forms to sign; no questions asked. My wage was to be exactly one-third of what I was earning as a teacher. My happiness was in inverse proportion to my wage. This was the first real decision that I had ever made alone — considering only my own feelings and needs, and giving myself the same chance as the next person in the street. Perhaps there was still a bit of hope left that I might become a person first, and an epileptic second.

It was bad luck that I was allotted to the bookshop's art department. Never having studied art history, even at school, the names of even the most famous artists, let alone the period during which they lived, were a mystery to me. The lady who ran the art department was quite a forceful charater. Her fingers were covered in rings, and her whole person dangled and clanked with odd bits of extravagant jewellery. Her age was a mystery, obscured by her red-dyed hair and her original make-up. She was greatly trusted by a large number of customers for her im-

116

mense knowledge of the art book world. No wonder she got so frustrated with me! She set me to dusting her precious (and often hideously expensive) art books. I climbed ladders and banged books together — the same books all through every day; because although I was so assiduous about it, the cleaner came every night and swept clouds of dust back on to the shelves again. The lowest shelves were coated in grit of various colours, depending upon which area of Australia the dust storms had come from that finally swirled in from the arcade and spent themselves in our bookshop. Australia is just a dusty place at the best of times.

My hands and clothes got filthy, I was doing hard menial work, the tendons in my legs were making me dizzy with pain from standing so long, the manageress kept scolding me like a mother hen, I was working long hours — and I felt freer and happier than at any other time in my life. This was me — a B A, Dip. Ed. world at-my-feet, on my hands and knees with the customers looking down their noses at my ignorance — in the last stages of ecstasy.

A certain amount of real physical tiredness is tremendously satisfying. It made me feel, then, as if I had actually achieved something every day — not a feeling I was used to from teaching, the factory or the non-combatants. Every evening I could sit on the back steps with Sloopy, knowing for a certainty that the evening was all mine. For as long as I could remember there had been a continual obligation to work after tea for an unspecified time: studying, preparation, marking and setting tests, which would go on for as long as my eyes could stay open. Now at last, some of the impulses to rush out and do things could be followed up. I planted butter beans and ranunculi, got out my guitar and songbooks, went to typing lessons; for the first time in years I was able to thoroughly enjoy talking to strangers leaning over their gates — a common Australian pastime when the heat of the day is over.

Such a sudden return of forgotten happiness and freedom should, I reasoned, have led to an immediate withdrawal of epileptic seizures. It did not. I had a greater number of *grand mals* that year than during the previous one. One day, my aunt came to visit me, and I must have had a fit as she drove away. I found myself in the dusk, lying on the back lawn, covered in prickles from the burr-grass, and red with mosquito bites. It was hard to face the fact of a fit alone at first. It was not sympathy I needed, so much as reassurance. But on the good side, it did give me ample time to sleep it off and recover completely.

To my great surprise I was still having *petit mals* at work. Yet I had been perfectly certain that all minor attacks would be finished with, along with my weekday dread. I had expected a much more dramatic change with this particular new start. An even greater surprise, though, was the simple fact that nobody noticed the *petit mals*. The superior art lady presumed I would be an ignoramus for at least a few months, so she expected me to look blank occasionally. As for her equally formidable customers, they prided themselves on their extreme patience with new shop assistants. So, when, after a question like 'Have you got the new Rembrandt collection in yet?' I appeared confused and uncomprehending, they stood there like perfect pictures of Job, even if I had it in my hand.

After a few such instances of embarrassment, I began to understand everybody's attitude. They were expecting me to be stupid, at least some of the time. Such an assumption made me extremely angry initially; until now I had always been expected to perform. But it did help, ultimately. Other people's acceptance of my hesitation in this job must have reached my sub-conscious, for the result was a remarkable improvement in my recovery time from *petit mals*. Also, I became less likely to have them consecutively, less likely to let them panic me into T L E, less vulnerable to the dangers of T L E, which was just as well, working in such a busy city and having to commute by train. And all this improvement was due to a simple psychological reaction not to extra drugs or to trick cyclists.

Customers always expect a bookseller to be a walking

dictionary/encyclopedia. Of necessity, I learned plenty of words and names in the next few weeks and was eventually informed enough to give guided tours of the illustrious and illustrated art department. But I was not learning the mechanics of the trade, and so I was pleased when one day I was transferred to the technical department under the guidance of a man with thirty years' experience as a bookseller.

Nobody in the shop had been told about my health record, but somehow it did not take long for my new manager, Mr Webb, to guess. He did not let on that he knew for some time. Perhaps he had watched me during *petit mals* and compared my appearance with that of a friend whose medical record he did know about. Perhaps he had wondered why someone with my qualifications was working as a shop assistant. But his suspicions did not change his opinion of me one bit. He watched me enthusiastically sorting out the mysteries of that varied department and he decided to train me.

We started having an extended morning tea-break in the Ceylon Tea Room, where he plied me with huge bowls of tea and passionfruit pavlova, gradually unfolding his extensive knowledge of 'the trade' and answering all my questions about everything that happened in the shop — right, wrong or indifferent. Here, then, was something that I could really believe in and work for, without fear of bureaucratic oppression. More importantly, someone actually believed in me at last, thought me worth teaching. I would have learned to be an undertaker if only to be accorded such esteem.

When I finally got up enough courage to tell the family, they wrote me off all over again. All that time and money wasted on an expensive education. They knew I should never have gone to university, knew I should have been sensible, sober and resigned from the start. Now look where it had got me! But my eccentric aunt and uncle thought it was a fabulous idea and encouraged me to stick to it. They had always accepted the possibility of me being a bit of a misfit — why did I want so desperately to change my nature? And 'misfit' does not automatically mean 'bad'. Moreover, the book trade was full of people who had failed in some profession and gravitated towards this one, which is demanding but does not try to mould people into a certain shape. 'Eccentrics Anonymous' it could be called. Here was one profession where I would not stick out like a sore toe — everyone else did too!

The large room in my flat was warmed by an old-fashioned, fluted gas heater. There were no protective bars and no fireguard. It was my habit to sit up late at night on an ancient, leather pouffé (which somebody's grandfather must have brought back from the Middle East after the War) and read, or just gaze into the flickering flames with their comforting flame noise. Sloopy would lie there too. One particular night, only three weeks after moving departments, I was leaning over the fire — more for comfort and restfulness than for warmth — and I had an epileptic fit. I must have fallen straight on to the brittle fluting and broken it with my face, but the fire did not go out. It was a miracle that I woke up at all, because I felt no pain. But I did wake. Luckily I was wearing a woollen jumper, which had resisted the flames (a man-made fibre would not have done so). Gradually, I returned to semi-consciousness and rolled around the floor as always. Then, crying with the pain in my fingers, I staggered into the kitchen to hold them under the cold tap. The only other pain was in my shoulder. But things did not feel right. Being in the usual fuzzy state after a *grand mal*, I could not work out exactly what was wrong, but something insisted that I should go and see my mother. Having no idea of the time, I thought that a reasonable enough request, so I walked out into the night and went home. It was only about two and a half miles. I banged on the fly-wire screen of the front door with the palms of my hands, moaning a little.

When my mother opened the door, well after midnight, she saw a sight which made her knees collapse under her. I must have looked pretty awful — face covered in white ash and already swelling; the hair on the right side gone and also, apparently, the ear; neck dripping with clear body fluid; pink jumper burnt and gaping, fingers wealed. The adrenalin having done its vital work, I collapsed inside the house. My mother rang the same G P who had seen me after the first fit. He was there in ten minutes. During one of the brief moments of consciousness, I heard him say that he must see where it had happened. We went back to the flat and found all the doors open, lights on and the gas fire burning away with a gaping hole in it. The sight was enough to make even this experienced doctor shudder. He has always marvelled at my miraculous escape. I was admitted to hospital immediately with shock, third-degree burns to face, head and hands, plus less serious burns in other places.

Nature, I have said, is kind. Burns are reputedly the most painful of all injuries. Yet I did not feel any pain in my face at all, only in the less serious burns on neck and shoulder. I was in a merciful state of complete shock. There was no pain for the next five weeks, which I spent quite passively and happily in hospital. Our G P had ordered me a room to myself and a cot-bed with sides, in case of a further fit. This rather annoyed me as I had to ask to get out of bed.

There was no mirror in the room and I never thought to ask for one. The burns must have made me look rather dreadful; my father came once to visit me, but not again. I even remember his look of horror and disbelief, he believed I would have ugly scarring for life — poor man, he had come on the second day when the swelling was at its height.

The flames had missed my eyes by one-eighth of an inch.

Three fingers were burned to the bone. I could see the bone every time they were dressed. My face looked pretty hopeless so the doctor decided to do an experiment with it. For five days the nurses sprayed on an anti-bacterial preparation (burns are very easily infected) which also caused a hard shell to form across my face, head and fingers. The lesser burns were treated with a pungent, yellow gauze. On the sixth day, the doctor came into my room dressed in green operating gear and followed by a surgical nurse and trolley. No warning! He lay me down and cut the shell off like a mask.

He had noticed in my records a fortunate tendency to heal quickly. That is why he tried this new idea first, rather than go through the excruciating and lengthy business of skin grafts. He covered the new, fragile flesh with what must have been a very valuable ointment — cortisone cream. Cortisone was being cautiously experimented with at the time. It was found to contain extremely useful properties for the treatment of arthritis and nerve ailments, and to stimulate skin growth after burns. It was a sort of miracle drug, except that its long-term effects were unknown. My skin responded like a peach in full bloom. The newly restored face was presentable to the world within five weeks; only my ear would require an operation.

Seven years later I still bear the scars of the price I paid for independence. But they are not unsightly (most people cannot even tell) and I was spared much additional agony. I don't even remember them now, when I look in the mirror. My hands do what they always did.

Shortly before I left the hospital, the nurses asked if I would speak to another girl with burns. She was also an epileptic and had had a fit under the shower. As she fell, she had knocked the cold tap, turning it off — and boiling water was pouring all over her body for about six minutes. Although she lived in a special hostel for epileptics, nobody had come to find her until it was too late. Her face was untouched but from neck to waist her skin was purple and wrinkled — it was especially bad on the sensitive part underneath her arms. This girl had been in hospital for almost a year while skin-grafts were done and she recovered from the shock of third degree burns. The blessing of shock had eliminated much initial pain for her also. She was still smiling.

It had been peaceful in the hospital, lying in bed and watching the winter sunlight on the square of gums at the front; seeing husbands come to collect wives with new babies; feeling safe. I had no anxieties about the future or about what I would look like when it was all over. Where my serenity came from I do not know. Perhaps I had developed a strong resilience by that time.

My mother, who had never failed a single visiting hour despite the agony my appearance must have given her, rang the bookshop and, under my directions, begged them to keep the job open. My dear old manager, guessing the truth and still believing in my future, had pleaded for me, so the job was waiting.

During subsequent treatment, the G P told me that such a violent shock could either make or break me. He said it for a warning, but I interpreted his words as a real sign of hope. I certainly had not gone all to pieces, so maybe things would go the other way. The conviction became strong in me that this fit was going to be the last, the very last.

There was, at least, an astonishing transformation of attitude. The process had probably already begun when I decided, first to go it alone in a flat and second, to leave teaching. Those were my decisions. But this fit had acted just like severe shock-treatment. It was the turning point in my life, both as an epileptic and as a person. I gave a great kick to the barriers separating me from the rest of the world. If that was the worst that could happen to me then I would never be scared to do anything alone again. And being alone left me free to find out about myself, to learn to like this self and then, maybe, to present a new and infinitely more assured person to others.

My entire outlook and philosophy changed. That miserable, ragged, baby owl of the folk song, who had spent so many years knocking about in the dark, was suddenly emerging into the glorious sunlight. The transition had nearly killed it, but there it was, gasping at all the new possibilities.

Back at work I told everyone that there had been a gas leak which made me pass out. This was readily accepted for at the time, Australia was changing from coal gas to natural gas. Several disastrous mistakes had been made, especially on older stoves and heaters. If I looked very bad, nobody said anything. In fact, some good things even came of those scars — for instance, I changed my hairstyle to cover the burns a bit, and it suited me; I also stopped wearing make-up.

There was a huge department store in the city which gave free advice and demonstrations to people with 'interesting beauty problems'. I was always a beauty problem, but now I had a real excuse. So I went out one lunch-time looking like Miss Muggs, had Monsieur Michel restyle my hair to alleviate the top half of the beauty problem, then went to the ground floor where Madame Michot covered the other half with various splodges of brown, white, red and blue — very patriotic. It was this last operation which, as it took three quarters of an hour, put me off make-up for ever. Although Madame did make me look rather smashing, I was too scared to smile in case my face literally cracked.

One other battle was still to be fought. I was determined to maintain my hard-won independence, so I went straight back to the flat, despite my mother's understandable entreaties — back to Sloopy, those twenty-one rose bushes, the potato patch, and a brand new fireguard.

13

It was during the following twelve months that a small article appeared in the Melbourne morning newspaper, the *Sun*. Headed 'Epilepsy is a Symptom; not a Disease', it was written by the newspaper's family doctor and was likely to be read by half a million people. The message, for Australia, was fairly advanced: epileptics are worth employing, are 'no different from you and me', are not touched by God or inhabited by devils. I hope a lot of people besides my mother (who showed me the cutting) read it, and benefited by it. Alas, there was also a lot of bad information in the article, such as a tendency to rate heredity high in the possible causes, to suggest that it was probably not a good idea for epileptics to have children, and that most epileptics become incontinent during fits. Comparing it with the most recent lay book on the subject, Burden and Schurr, *Understanding Epilepsy* (Crosby Lockwood, 1976), I find it annoying to say the least — but at least this document had described, in black and white, what many people were afraid even to discuss. A seed was sown in my mind, just at the right time, from the article. There was nothing, nothing to be ashamed of.

Part of taking my chances as just another person meant resolving not to tell a soul about the epilepsy. It meant not having my grand excuse to cushion the inevitable blows of disappointment and failure. The resolution held good at work, because I feared losing my job — the first job I had ever really wanted to keep. But I found it difficult to communicate with fellow workers on a normal, conversational level; some well-laid intellectual snobbery prevented me from discussing football, popgroups, the world situation, fashions or the price of fish. At twenty-three, it did rather seem as if I was to become a confirmed old maid, set in my ways and intolerant of others.

Tolerance and patience are not among my glowing virtues. As I sat moodily in the cheerless lunchroom which smelt of machine-made coffee and was too hot to think in properly, a painful awareness began to dawn on me. I had never been or done anything to anybody for them to care about me. It was, therefore, not me who required other people's sympathy and patience, but everyone else who required mine. Major revelation!

About this time, Liz returned from working for two years as a jillaroo (female Australian cowboy) in Queensland. She was now teaching autistic children, an exhausting job in every way, and she often spent her free days at the flat. We would go trampolining or ten-pin bowling, and she would make carrot soup on the tiny, gas stove.

I began to look forward greatly to her visits – to talk and to listen, to laugh and commiserate, to go out together or stay at home and listen to music, to get enthusiastic about things – and to be silent. I was twenty-four, just beginning to learn and enjoy the basic psychology of human friendship.

With that, I got up enough confidence to join the local choral society, and soon became the treasurer. We had only two concerts a year, a paucity of tenors and few really good singers. But it was fun – and we shared our enjoyment of singing with the old people in nearby homes and hospitals. Also, we sang carols at the large mental hospital near Melbourne. There were several wards that we could not go near, only singing outside the barred windows, but we could hear sounds of recognition and appreciation from these unfortunate people. Here was another revelation for me. For so long I had been morbidly occupied with my own illnesses, real and imagined. But these people were genuinely ill. The lesson came as a booster to the shock I received from the burns shock. I resolved to banish all defeatism as of that Christmas, if it was humanly possible.

Apparently it was not humanly possible. The old persecution complex remained and I was often in what looked to outsiders, like the sulks, for weeks. But it was more, complex to pinpoint than as just sulking. It was, more, a temporary withdrawal from the world due to a renewed fear of people. At such times my face would resume the hard, set mask that had begun in my first job at the hospital. It was like being stuck in a big hole of my own making and I just had to wait until I had enough strength to climb out of it again. Meanwhile the perpetual lump of misery was lodged in my throat, and I would fly home to Sloopy each day, aching for those lone hours when I could throw off the mask and swallow the misery, smiling, laughing and talking with her.

Even Mr Webb, my manager and teacher and friend, was not able to shake me out of these moods. I would speak to him for days on end, only in an official capacity, with pursed lips and frigid face. He would smile a little sadly, sigh, shake his head and wait. He was the most patient man I could ever hope to meet.

Mr. Webb was shortish, stoutish, baldish, oldish. His hair had once been red, his eyes had often smiled, and his face was deeply lined. His marriage had been wrecked years before and the children were taken away, which must have grieved him — he was a fatherly man. He was inclined to get drunk when things were not going right and his stomach would bulge over the worn belt of his trousers. It was easy to tell that he did for himself, just by looking at his sporadic attempts to dress properly. Mr. Webb did not have much to say. In fact, he was, it might be said, an unremarkable person, a dull little man. But that was not so. He was a champion.

The morning breaks of tea and pavlova with him contined. (If you don't know what pavlova is, grab the nearest Australian girl, who will tell you that marriages in Melbourne are made or marred, not on the girl's figure, brains or humour, but on her 'pavs'.) I'd levelled with Mr Webb about the reasons for the burns; he had accepted the explanation as something he already knew. To my joyful amazement he dismissed it all as irrelevant to my future and so our training sessions were resumed with a new dimension of absolute trust.

We had some great times together, unlikely pair that we were. I only realized how close we indeed became with the shock of his death shortly after I left Australia. He had been just like a father to me. He even taught me to laugh again. The most hilarious time I remember with him was, oddly enough, on the day of the Great Flood.

We had been having a terrible drought — even by Melbourne standards. One day in late February, all the rain we should have had over the past five months decided to fall between 1.30 and 4.30 p.m. Four inches. Now that is all very well, except that the storm was centred in the city itself.

Melbourne is built on the Yarra River. (The Sydneyites maintain that the Yarra is Melbourne's only claim to fame, being the only river in the world that flows upside-down, with the mud at the top.) Right next to the river is the big commuter train station, Flinders Street, with thirteen platforms. One of its two front entrances, where all the commuters go in or out, depending on the time of day, and where all the tramlines from the university and beyond end, is a big subway in Elizabeth Street, Our shop was on this major shopping street, which had been built over a dry creek bed a hundred years before. The street is in the very centre of the city, and all the other streets go steeply down to it and steeply up again. So, when four inches of rain fall in three hours, and the storm water drains are blocked in ten minutes, Elizabeth Street will revert to its original form — a tributary river of the Yarra.

By 2.30 p.m. the main station had been closed. The streams of people had been replaced by streams of water which filled the subways right up to the 'Please Do Not

Spit' level. The cars parked in Elizabeth Street were now floating randomly down towards the station, crashing into each other. Even when the water was four feet deep some people tried to cross the street — the single-minded Australian cannot believe that anything will stop him. One man near us took off his shoes and trousers, then swam across the street with a sort of side-stroke, holding his garments in the same hand as an ineffectual black umbrella.

Meanwhile all trading had ended as we watched the waters rise in disbelief — and with some considerable amusement. A small knot of refugee customers were marooned in the raised paperback department because, to our amazement, the water was coming through the doors. There was no question of closing them against the surge of water. The flood washed across the ground floor like a slow-motion movie and my relief that the technical department's basement area would not be touched was short-lived. The water swept down the stairs, first in a trickle and finally in the most exciting waterfall that you can ever hope to see in the basement of a bookshop.

Mr Webb and I were wading around with our shoes off, trying to save the stock on the lower shelves and having a real field-day, despite missing our afternoon tea. Mr. Webb was a quick thinker. As the waters roared down into the lower basement, where they finally rose to within three inches of the electricity fuses, you might have found him behind the central pillar with a bucket of dirty water. He was dunking all the previously damaged or old stock, and even old editions which we could not get rid of. He gave a wink and I was in on the act immediately, bringing him all the old stock that had plagued me for months by its very dusty presence.

We had a grand writing-off session and a presentable figure to produce for the insurance inspectors. The art department had been saved by its loftiness, but the Ceylon Tea Room was awash for several weeks. Then followed a magnificent Flood Sale, and every other shop within cooee of the flood had one too. There was a Christmas atmosphere, that hot February in Melbourne. Everybody had to buy something salvaged from the Great Flood. The only people who were not smiling were the insurance brokers, and they could afford it.

They say an epileptic fit is rather like a stroke. After a stroke, people often have difficulty with speech and also with writing, although the thought processes themselves are perfectly agile. For me one small problem, apart from *petit mal*, was the realization that my speech was not all that it should be and was not improving. While thoughts were buzzing around in my head as usual, while I was able to assess and act upon a situation quite smartly, it was difficult to communicate this understanding or interpret arguments into anything but a simple, rather lame, string of words.

It always helps me to know the cause of such developments and I found it even interesting to learn that the lesion on my brain was almost certainly in the lower-middle half of the brain — the area that deals with speech; that part of my brain function was affected nearly all the time to some degree. If you look at a 'brain-map', it will be apparent that the part dealing with speech is slightly above and forward of the ears — just the place where those forceps might have been placed during a more frantic moment at my birth.

In some ways, this has turned out to be a blessing in disguise. For someone as rash and opinionated as I am, deliberation before speech is a very good idea. Besides, the face can be expressive: smiles, frowns, nods, grimaces are all part of an international language. This speech problem has grown and continues to plague me at times. Friendships carried on by letter are so much more successful then confrontation relationships. Also, having people around for days, or even hours, exhausts and confuses me. It is the conversations I suppose. However much I enjoy people's company, even the simplest question requires an answer, and before answering, a decision must be made.

When someone says, 'How are You?' there are thousands of possible answers. It might be a polite introduction or a genuine inquiry into my health. Should I say: 'Very well, thank you,' or 'How are you?'; 'Awful! I've got a rotten cold' (state of health) or 'miserable. My cat's run away' (state of mind); 'On top of the world', 'Ready for anything'; or even such enigmatic phrases as 'Well I never!' and 'How do you think?' The brain-computer has to do an almighty dive to find the most suitable answer and come out with it at half a second's notice. My brain tends to panic and grab for the responses about 'boyfriends' when I need the one across the way marked 'grandmothers'. Then I spend the next five minutes trying to explain the mistake away.

The result is nearly always a minor seizure within about an hour. Strangely enough, this does not seem to hold true for job interviews; I really shine at those. Perhaps it is the knowledge that they have no preconceived idea about what I might say. But generally, long and intense conversations are not ultimately successful. When it finally comes to the necessity of answering a complex question involving a large number of factors, my brain-computer makes a frenzied dash around all the necessary corridors, collects all the various bits of information required — and promptly blacks out with the weight and import of it all.

There is a certain amount of psychology involved in the sacred disease but each of us has to discover that for himself. It we give in to the little devil, he will use the victory to make life a burden. But if we can tell him to get lost, and mean it with all our energies, there is no doubt that he does, at least, go to the back of the theatre and only taunt us when we look at him. My little devil must have been thoroughly flummoxed. Ater what he thought to be such a victory on his home-ground, fire, the only result was that for the first time since our acquaintance, I really had no fear of him at all.

Three months after recovering from the burns I had

another bad fit, but its psychological effects on me were negligible. I was crossing a main trunk road at peak hour and woke up in hospital. Fortunately, although I had fallen in the middle of the road, no car had even touched me. And by this time my morale was such that I walked out of the casualty department and took a train home. Epilepsy was going to have to step down as a major factor in my life. I got rid of the bracelet.

Although I had worn a bracelet or a 'Medic Alert' disc around my neck for so many years, I cannot think of one occasion when it was useful. Even during the *grand mal* on the main road, people thought that I was either a drug addict or, for some reason, drunk or a diabetic. Strangers, even enlightened ones, confronted with the brief drama of a fit are too worried about the safety of the patient to begin searching for a possible identification tag — even if it occurs to them to look for such a thing. Those concerned with epileptics may not realize just how demoralizing it is when they try to persuade all of us to carry such identification. Every few minutes of the day, even subconsciously with the jingle on the chain, we are reminded that we are different.

Morale is immensely important in epilepsy and now I was learning to consider myself as not so very different after all. Once the identification disc was thrown away, my relief was amazing. Living without the tag and taking my chances, I found it much easier to go for days and weeks without remembering my special status. That made it easier to treat myself more severely, stop making excuses and start making greater attempts to succeed in those areas of life where I could be found wanting.

With the advent of efficient drug-control, the epileptic's lot has changed completely. Not once have I mentioned 'the sufferer', but only 'the patient'. Agreed, there is something physically wrong with us but apart from the immediate after-effects of a *grand mal*, we don't really suffer at all.

As a child I was asthmatic, had pneumonia and was

weak and spindly. I would walk down the street to the shops with my mother and listen to the matriarchs of the community leaning over their gates, wagging their knotty fingers at me and assuring my mother in stentorian tones, 'You'll never raise that child!' That made me so angry that I determined to grow up and show them all. When my grandfather, trying to make me eat boiled vegetables, would poke my belly and say, 'Plenty of room in there yet. Eat some more,' I would submit only because of the old ladies' warnings.

Since becoming an epileptic I have been strong and absurdly healthy, enjoying hard physical work and sports like moutaineering. I rarely have even a cold. Compare this lot with the arthritic, the migraine sufferer, people with neuralgia, stomach ulcers and other constant aches; even the diabetic must choose between a rigid diet and daily injections. Compare it also with the fear of people with heart disease or any form of cancer. These people really do suffer although they have not the added fear of rejection by society. We have that instead. I know what I would prefer.

With Mr Webb's continual encouragement came a growing sense of purpose. Despite the frequent bouts of loneliness, life was appearing to become meaningful at last. New possibilities and greater horizons opened and loomed respectively until I was dizzy with excitement. Mr Webb said he had taught me everything he knew and that I must now go to Great Britain for further experience. Fantastic thought — go to Britain! The wonderland of Dickensian London, Hardy's Dorset, everybody's Cambridge, Agatha Christie's wealthy murders and — The Bronte moors. Australians had not yet discovered their own excellent literature. We were brought up on a diet of undiluted ancestorworship which makes everyone feel at home the minute they step off the boat.

But for me to do it. Me with all my . . . . Well, with all

these . . . . Well, exactly why shouldn't I go after all? Mr Webb lovingly nurtured the idea he had planted. Nor was he the only one to pamper it. My eccentric aunt and uncle also thought it was a great idea. They did not say, 'You can't travel alone and so far away because you're an epileptic and need shielding and a quiet life.'

I finally made the big decision, to attempt the great adventure with all its possibilities for success — or failure. Suddenly there was a good supply of mental energy to tackle all the details of how and when. For too long I had been living within a narrow set of rules saying, 'You can't do this — most other people do, but not you.' Lots of people go travelling, and alone too. But it was hard work for me to cut through the great tangle of 'rules for me' to see the possibilities behind emerge.

Perhaps a pioneering spirit born of six generations of squatters and a thirst for adventure had now been roused. I took a job as a waitress at night, typed a friend's M Sc thesis and started feverishly saving up. Ham sandwich for 17¢? No — jam sandwich for 7¢ plus another one in London. New dress for $20? No — alter an old one and spend a week in Scotland instead. Thus it was that I reasoned myself across ten thousand miles of sea while working on the basic wage.

That job as a waitress did not last long — the restaurant owner kept taking my tips. So I got a job as a cashier in the most exclusive eating place in Melbourne. The pay was better and I got fed like a princess every night. Some of the friendly wine waiters would bring me extra desserts and after-dinner mints, as well as endless cups of real coffee and such perks as cherry liqueurs. That was quite an experience. The whole enormous idea, plus all its consequences was quite an experience. Admittedly, Mr Webb had had to give me a push before my mind would even entertain such a notion as taking two jobs or being a waitress. I did not tell the restauranteurs that I was an epileptic. Why should I? I honestly did not believe that there was going to be another fit.

But there was considerable opposition to the flight of this ugly duckling. Never having left the sunny shores themselves (in common with everyone for three generations back), the family simply could not understand why I wanted to go to a dismal, foggy, smoggy, unfriendly country which was by all accounts plain broke. Didn't we live in the land of milk and honey? I had not a single friend or relation to appeal to or fall back on or advise me in Britain (thank God, I thought, what a fabulous place it must be). How could I ever get proper medical attention over there? What if . . . what if I had a fit amongst strangers? Strangers are people. Even British strangers. Besides I was not going to have another fit. Hitting new heights of optimism I took my hard-earned money and booked the cheapest ticket available. Doing three jobs at once had not killed me — it had done the opposite.

On 7 October 1972, nine trunks, three months' supply of pills, several thousand disgruntled migrants, and a hopeful me left for England.

14

It was, admittedly, a bit sad seeing the lights of Melbourne growing smaller as the huge ship steamed slowly out to the open sea. But I felt no regret. Mr Webb came early to say his good-byes with some beautiful flowers. Saying little, I knew he meant much — there was much encouragement and some little pride in his bearing, as well as some sadness. This was the very thing he had always wanted to do himself, but somehow never got around to it. He had even bought his ticket once. In spirit, he was coming with me. A telegram came to say, 'Happy Christmas — letter follows'. The letter never came and he died of a brain haemorrhage soon afterwards.

My friend Liz could not come, being two thousand miles away. Dad had already said good-bye, but my mother came. She was naturally very upset. But to me the psychological necessity of getting away from all possible props was paramount. So far I had not risked total independence. There had always been someone fairly near to whom I could run when necessary. What I needed was a real testing ground where I would be thrown right back on my own resources if life started to get bumpy. It was the only way to find out if I could be truly independent — or if I would need Watchers for the rest of my life.

Ours was a large cabin, way below the waterline. I shared it with two failed migrants and one Bolivian. The English ladies' greatest ambition was to return to West Bromwich and eat proper chips. All the pressure of packing and good-byes over, I began to relax. Four days out of port, I had a full-scale *grand mal* during breakfast. At that stage people were still going to bed in time to get up for breakfast, and a very few had reached the stage of staying up for breakfast and then going to bed. So I must have alarmed quite a lot of people. I was dragged into the ship's hospital and given an injection. I dread to think what it was — both doctor and nurse could only speak Greek and I could only speak Strine. So I pulled myself together much quicker than is usually possible and wobbled or crawled my way back to the cabin.

I was dismayed, no, positively angry at this new exhibition of strength by my little devil. The old fear that everybody must have seen the fit and judged me accordingly, returned. That was definitely not how I had planned things. An enormous passenger liner is a closed shop of circulating gossip. People have so much time on their hands that their tongues are liable to work overtime. I did not realize, for a few weeks, that they are really only interested in each other's sex lives.

I began to spend some of the eternal leisure hours in the Marine Bar with a group of young Aussies who were not so much going to England as running away from Australia. The returning British migrants avoided the Australians on board at all costs. We had nothing to do but swap gossip for five weeks; but as my Great Secret was already out, I was a listener — until it became unendurably boring. Could it have been possible that all this soul-searching, this self-pity under pretence of reason would have been my lot also, had it not been for that *grand mal* near Wellington? Certainly the fit postponed the start of my social life. But at least it saved me from those awful shipboard romances which flare up during a tango and are consummated on deck under a starry sky. All very well until the destination is reached and the world gets back into perspective.

It was nice to have a complete rest — for about a week. Some of us performed a melodrama in which I played the chivalrous young man. The same group performed a revue based on ship board life, for which I wrote all the words to the songs. So I did find myself being able to participate in any worthwhile activities, despite the initial shame of that very public *grand mal*, with its accompanying anger and frustration. People were not bothering about it nearly so much as I feared. Being at leisure for the first time since becoming an epileptic, I was well able to assess people's reactions to such a display in a fully social situation. As we lazed around the decks and Marine Bar, I came to an amazing conclusion. It did not matter to them.

Nobody was looking oddly at me; I was quickly included in all activities despite my shyness. Everybody showed a genuine interest in the mechanics of an epileptic fit. They asked lots of questions which I found myself answering with as much disinterest as if I were my own neurologist. Then, just as if we had been solving the world's problems, the subject was dismissed and others were substituted. They had forgotten! The results of my close scrutiny of the events did not sink in immediately, but that journey was invaluable to my self-confidence. Apparently, people could accept the fact of epilepsy in me as easily as the fact of my big feet.

We reached Southampton, rounding the Isle of Wight too early for almost everybody on the ship to see their first English coast. The farewell ball had been a lengthy, emotional affair. I reverently partook of my first meal in England, sitting in a comfortable old Rover with two of the landed gentry, on a suitably foggy November afternoon. The murky weather, the gloom of Savernake Forest, thrilled me nearly as much as the homemade, cold pork pie (unheard of in Australia), and lukewarm milk coffee which these folk had prudently packed for the journey. Being a bit old-fashioned, my hosts avoided motorways like the latest plague, but my first view of these phenomena, as we passed over them in the fog was exciting beyond description. Such things I had only heard of, read about, seen pictures of. But there it was — a British motorway, flowing out of the darkness on one side and back in again on the other. *Nous sommes arrivés* (in my best Australian accent).

I dread to think just how many times up until this point I had started out with a completely new set of people and circumstances, then promptly sat back and expected everything to be transformed. It had always misfired, mostly through my own mismanagement but with a bit of bad luck on the side. I did it again.

The people who collected me at Southampton were parents of a girl on the boat. They had a grand estate in Herefordshire and were the soul of kindness, typical of the fast-disappearing set of country people who used to mean 'the English' for me. As a guest in their home, I soon got used to four meals a day instead of three, and I went on long walks, climbing the bare trees, the better to see and luxuriate in the scenery — the reality of a dream come true. There were beautiful coal fires every evening — another new experience. They wanted to know all about the ship, their daughter (who had remained in Brazil), and me. While I was discussing university, bookselling, Australia and cattle-breeding they thought me just a nice, ordinary girl whom they were pleased to entertain.

But then my face slipped. The climate changed when I started telling my tales of woe and epilepsy. Why did I feel the need to tell them at all? Why could I not be the ordinary person which I had long been striving for? Perhaps I had done something rather scandalous and wanted to get back into their good graces. It was certainly not the fact of the epilepsy which altered their view but my unfair appeal to their sympathies. The little veneer of confidence collapsed, and I was back to the 'I'm-an-epileptic-so-you've-got-to-be-nice-to-me' stage. Two years in the flat had not taught me so much after all.

This is the way it had always worked. Ready to chat about any subject concerning myself, I was leaving out a whole half of human conversation, the 'How about you?' half. As soon as I stopped being the centre of attention there came a fear of rejection. Then I would desperately play that last, well-worn card — epilepsy. The look-for reaction never lasted long, but I could not understand why it went. All I knew was that something was wrong and it must be my fault. I craved people's acceptance. I was still going the wrong way about getting it.

The frightful stories of British poverty we had heard made us feel it was advisable to bring a complete survival kit — hence my nine trunks. Bedding, cutlery, china, saucepans, tea-strainers and teapot, biscuit barrel and a year's supply of condensed milk along with many offerings of woolly socks and vests from the family were packed in those trunks. From what the Australian media said, I gathered that virtually no items could be expected to be freely available in Britain at all.

I was looking forward to living in a broom cupboard with a candle, blissfully gazing through the cracks in the wall, which let the snow in a bit. When I arrived I found it was indeed possible to buy a can-opener with a small effort; the people looked disappointingly plump and were certainly clothed, albeit with the aid of Marks and Sparks. I could have left my year's supply of everything at home.

My first real autumn — the grandeur of bare trees black against a setting sun, darkness at 4.30 p.m., a wild squirrel, toadstools with spots, fog. My first real ruined castle — Ludlow, with a football match far below, followed by the new experience of toasted tea-cake in town. Then my first Cambridge landlady, who simply did not believe in bicycles, booksellers or boyfriends. Baths once a week, ten pence each. Old fluted gas-fire, with a fireguard. A gorgeous view across the Cam, Jesus Green and the crooked rooftops. Everything was magic. I was not to have another *grand mal* for a year, a record for me.

I had received a provisional job in a bookshop in Cambridge, provided I did not have two heads, or something worse. When filling in the application form I came to the space labelled 'Health Record' and prickled with apprehension. I considered putting either 'Yes please' or'No thank you'. As a compromise I wrote 'childhood asthma' and left it at that. It was not the first time and will not be the last that I strategically ignore such a question. Too many employers have too many preconceptions about the word 'epileptic'. Nothing will convince me that an epileptic with the possibility of one day-fit per year while at work is not a safer working bet than people with three-day migraines, susceptibility to changes in the weather, take-it-easyitis, long tea–breakivity, let's-have-a-gossipitis or very close veins. At least we are glad of the chance to work and are less liable to endanger our prospects with laziness or absenteeism. It is worth an employer's while to consider this. I entered the literature department of the large university bookshop with a clean bill of health and a clear conscience.

My silence on the subject continued. The only person in that organization who knew why I took all those pills was a young man who started taking me to his home for the new experience of Sunday dinners and generally kept me from feeling lonely without insisting on a passionate romance. I gave in to the strong temptation of telling Peter my secret, if only to relieve the strain of hiding it. Besides, it had always been hammered into me that I must let somebody working with me know, in case of a *grand mal*. There were several points to weigh up. Telling anybody always made me feel inferior and changed my personality in relation to the person I told. Ridiculous, but recognizably true, for me. Then there was the safety angle. If nobody knew, what could happen? Nobody knew on the ship, either, but I survived that *grand mal*. A bookshop is not a highly dangerous place in which to have a fit. There was nowhere in particular to fall. I was not afraid of having one there – so I would chance it. But Pete was the first person to whom I told my secret voluntarily, matter-of-factly and with no ulterior motives. He asked what all the pills were for. I told him. He became protective –but only to the degree that he would be with any girl

-- and considerate as well as a good friend.

If the autumn had been magic, then the winter was an orgy of wonderment. Living with three other girls and a resident landlady was not my idea of heaven but it took several months for the 'Hey, I'm in England!' feeling to wear off. The greatest excitement was the first time that I saw ice on the Cam, stood on it and cracked the nearby puddles with my shoes. And then my first snow. I went crazy with delight, whooping around on the bicycle, scattering staid old ducks and swans along the river banks.

Without knowing it, I was also becoming quite an entertaining phenomenon at the shop. 'Bumptious' is scarcely the word; I was more like a steamroller trying to dance like Zorba the Greek in my efforts to know everything, learn everything, be everything. The English smiled, laughed and looked on. I was excused on account of being a foreigner (an excuse which I still find very useful), accepted in spite of everything I did and said. The process of growing up should now be able to begin in earnest, about seven years later than it should have done. The scruffy owlet, thrown out alone into the light, was beginning to see, and was making a lot of comical fluttering in its attempts to walk like a sparrow and sing like a skylark.

It was necessary, soon, to register with a doctor. But I soon discovered that an ordinary G P cannot prescribe drugs for chronic ailments on a long-term basis, without the blessing of a specialist. Moreover, the most important drug for me, dilantin, was unknown — at least by its brand name. It was just good luck that my old pill bottle had a small label marked 'phenytoin sodium' and we were able to identify the stuff as epanoitin in Britain.

Then I had the brilliant idea that, since I was in the greatest country in the world for medicine, and within reach of a famous research hospital, I may as well ask the specialist if anything could be done for me. Perhaps there might have been some incredible breakthrough in the field of epilepsy that had not yet filtered down to the Antipodes. So an appointment with a neurologist at the famous Addenbrookes Hospital was made.

I was not a little surprised to find an Australian neurologist in the consulting room, and even more surprised when she told me, a bit sadly, in answer to my question as to the possibility of curing me, that the best place in the world for my complaint was — the Royal Melbourne Hospital. So there was nothing to be done. Dr Ebeling would have been the first to know of a cure, or a surer method of control. I had not really had any hopes, so I was not too disappointed. An E E G was done and the new drugs prescribed. What a pity! But . . . well . . . I don't think that I would have been brave enough for a fancy brain operation, anyway.

The neurologist advised me to join the British Epilepsy Association straight away. With no enthusiasm, I finally sent away and received several pamphlets, plus a large card which I was supposed to keep in my handbag. On it was printed 'I am an Epilpetic' in bold, black letters on a bright red background. I tried it for a few days. Every time I opened my bag for a handkerchief or purse, I could see those words flashing angrily out at me. I was appalled and dismayed. Who would be likely to open my bag to look for such a card if I did have a fit on the street? Goodness — it was twice as bad as the 'Medic Alert', because I was likely to read it twenty times a day! It would not take long to get brainwashed. I am an Epileptic. I am special . . . I am different . . . . I tore it up into little bits and threw it away.

Despite changing residences three times, I still could not get on with the communal life of bed-sitter existence and became unduly upset if I thought I was not going to get the prescribed eight hours' sleep. Why couldn't they keep quiet after 11 p.m.? Why couldn't they wash their dishes? Why didn't they leave me alone (or alternatively, come and talk to me)? Anyway, there was never any hot water left. Even at work I discovered that I had a remarkable capacity for rubbing people up the wrong way. Such actions as stamping one's feet at a general manager to stress one's point are simply not done in Britain. But still kept trying. There was obviously no compromise in ths new, emergent personality. What had happened to the long-awaited, all-pervading transformation? I could not see it. But there was one.

These people had no preconceptions about me at all, except the rather amusing view that they had of all Australians. Otherwise, it was a grand opportunity to become someone. I had to find an identity rather swiftly in order to present it to this rather reactionary, yet extraordinarily open-minded set of people. It turned out to be very different from the identity that had been laboriously salvaged from the remains left by the school children. But the basic material was inevitably the same. It was simply a matter of choosing the bits wisely and arranging them more sensibly.

It was during that beautiful year in idyllic Cambridge that I fell madly in love for the first time. Andy was born in London, brought up in Cambridge and his heart was all in sailing. He was happiest in a Thames barge or in a half-decker on the fens. I hope he is there now. It became a common and (I would imagine) amusing sight to see me flying around the bookshop yelling out 'Hey! I'm in love — I'm in love! Isn't it marvellous?' There was actually growing in me an ability to give love rather than to just soak it dry.

That was shortly after Andy saved my life. It was my second attempt to find a satisfactory bed-sitter. I had met him on the stairs, we had had supper together a few times and I had just told him of my epilepsy. This was a great stroke of luck because when he heard splashing and thrashing in the bathroom, he guessed what was happening. I had stupidly put the 'Engaged' latch on the door, one of the first 'Do Nots' for epileptics in bathrooms, but our Andy was undaunted. He got it open with a 2p piece. Without him, there was a good chance of me drowning, even though my survival instincts do seem to be especially strong. I often wonder how he felt, dragging a naked, dripping girl out of the bath. But that was not the only reason why we fell in love.

After a year, when the clash of cultures between a speak-your-mind Aussie and the status-quo Brits had resulted in some fine bursts of temper, things were getting a bit hot. Furthermore, I was finding it impossible to live on the minuscule wages offered, however little I tried to eat, so I considered changing jobs. It was just as well.

On the Saturday of the week before I was due to leave, when the shop was packed with customers, my little devil chose to put up a fight. It was now over a year since my last *grand mal* and the memory of what it was like had faded. I had all but forgotten the unbearable nausea and headache, the terrifying fear of death, the shame of what others had seen — and the dreadful frustration of having yet another epileptic fit when the belief had been so strong that the *grand mals*, at least, were done with. This one was a prolonged spectacular fit. As I writhed around on the floor (fortunately it had a good thick carpet), the managers were quite frightened and called an ambulance. I was in no condition to protest. There is the sort of risk we run if we decide not to tell our employers of the disability. It is not a physical risk — nobody can help at such a time — but the boss's confusion and possible anger could cost us our job. Personally, I believe that if we are worth keeping, they will keep us on anyway. It is much more difficult to get in than to stay in.

Peter told the bosses briefly and came with me in the ambulance. I had not recovered enough to know where I was or what was going on before I promptly had another fit. Poor Peter — although he had heard me speak of epilepsy, it must have given him a shock to actually see me during a fit. Later, when he was quite sure it would not hurt me to be told, he admitted that the spectacle was frightening and hard to rationalize because it looked much worse than it really was. It put him at a distance from me for some time, just as it had done with Liz at school, a distance caused by awe, fear for me and a feeling of helplessness, which my younger brother had already described.

Having a *grand mal* in front of a good friend can create difficulties, especially at the beginning of the relationship, before you have learned to value each other for your own particular qualities. But some epileptics prefer to get it over with so that both parties know where they stand. For someone having a *grand mal* every week or every month, it is probably better that way. It is amazing how quickly an ordinary person can dismiss and forget what might seem such an unfortunate event to us at the time. It is a matter of getting used to the idea of onlookers and not letting it make any difference in our attitudes towards them.

I will never know what effect that demonstration might have had on my job or my fellow-workers. Notice had already been given and I left for London a week later.

15

The job I had involved backroom work in bookselling — the mail-order department. The boss knew I was an epileptic; I told him at the interview. It was no longer any use trying to forget about it with British employers, because whenever they rang back to Cambridge for references, that is probably the first bit of unofficial information that they were given. The boss had another epileptic working on the switchboard and was not at all perturbed at the prospect of taking me on. Generally it was a happy place to work. Concern was rewarded with loyalty; commission was rewarded with harder work. If only all employers had this man's attitude, how easy it would be for us! Epileptics are still in a position to be grateful for work; we still need to work harder than the average person for less money, in order to retain a job and self-respect. This was the first job I had ever had where my employer knew my disability from the start and dismissed it as irrelevant. It brought a totally new dimension into my idea of work — specific knowledge that an employer could want me, including the epilepsy — because I was at last competing as an equal for positions in this career. No exceptions or conditions.

I have never thought it a very good idea to know too much about one's illnesses. It can lead to a morbid, self-preoccupation; a searching for symptoms which are not present and even a demand to know why they are not present. Although I had worked for three months in one of the most comprehensive medical book departments in Britain, it had simply not entered my head to go searching through the neurology section. But I became slightly

147

curious after the first interview with my new London specialist.

That was in the shining, new outpatients department of University College Hospital. The whole place runs like a quartz clock and I can never count on having a cup of tea for 2p while waiting for my appointment. Dr Stern seemed particularly interested in the number of T L E attacks I was having, and he put me straight on to garoin – a combination of epanoitin and phenobarb – which is supposed to work wonders in such cases. There was certainly a marked difference, even if it was only psychological. I began to feel bright-eyed and bushy-tailed and full of energy. But did I suffer from neuralgia? Yes, I suppose so; for many years I had suffered from 'face-ache' and was wryly amused when I solved the problem while studying for exams by tying a pair of tights around my chin and head. So the tegretol was increased. That should take care of the neuralgia.

What about my gums? Did I have trouble with them? No – what could he have meant? That is when I made the mistake of looking up a medical textbook, meant for doctors who are studying to be neurologists. I was appalled at the various sorts of symptoms that I might show, the reactions I might have to the drugs. No. I did not have swollen gums! And I had been taking phenytoin for ten years. There is no such thing as a general rule to any facet of epilepsy. I shut the book straight after that, and decided to leave all speculation to my specialist. Until he finds out, I would rather not know.

London. Mornings in the tube train. A layer of grime forms over your face after a couple of hours changing trains or racing the taxis around Aldwych or hanging on to a red bus as it swings along, making very little real headway. Unless you are a millionaire tourist, London is grim.

I moved seven times in four months and reluctantly settled for a half-finished room in an unfinished flat above a blue-movie club in Islington. The men came and went in dark glasses and grey macs. They went in one door for the film — that was the theory. Then they came to our door and applied for a date to practise — there had once been a brothel in the flat above that place!

I was on the minimum wage and after rent, fares and fuel bills, I had about £5 to live on. I didn't quite starve but it got close. An anti-starvation plan was required. I was not going to give up my new job so easily and I dared not ask for a rise, so I did the inevitable — became a barmaid four nights a week in order to eat enough to do two jobs.

Here follows a typical dialogue between my old self (call her Queen Victoria) and my new, aspiring self (a bit like Barbra Streisand, with any luck).

Q V: My dear girl! You know very well you can't be a ... a barmaid!

B S: Really? Why not?

V: Well, dear, it's just not respectable. Besides, if you must know, you're just too plain.

B: Beauty is in the eye of the beholder.

V: Perhaps — I can just imagine what sort of beholders you'll have in a public house. But even more important — you won't get enough sleep.

B: I can make do. I've had two jobs going before — and thrived on it.

V: A further thing — you've never been inside a public bar. You wouldn't know where to start.

B: It won't take long to learn — millions of other girls have done it.

V: Silly girl — you'll be on your feet all day and all night.

B: Yes — and I'll get a whole new look at a whole new set of people.

V: All right — what if all this extra strain and activity increases the number of fits? What if you have a fit in the bar?

B: I won't.

Islington is not the most savoury of neighbourhoods. It is on the murky old Regent's Canal, the streets are filthy, the parks are ill-kept and there are too many people per square yard. It is a neighbourhood of crooks and men on 'the lump', of beaten wives and stolen cars and broken windows and evidence of dogs all along the pavement.

When I worked at the Island Queen it was run by a tubby ex-boxer who ate three steaks a day and could turn out troublemakers with a finger and thumb. And there were troublemakers. There was plenty of money, too. Sticky rolls of fivers would appear to pay for a ten-man round or placate a wife who had been told to shut up and go home. Nor were they only buying bitter.

It was busy, almost frantic at times — with men four-deep around the bar, all yelling, half-drunk, the juke-box playing 'Candle in the Wind' and the sound of smashed glass. There were three wooden ladies, larger than life, sitting on stools above the bar, dressed in lace curtains and sequins like call girls, with their carved legs at all angles. I never did see the connection between them and the Queen. It was a man's pub. There were always at least four girls behind the bar. We did not have time to look pretty and chat up the customers. It was all sweat. I loved it. I loved walking home at midnight around those dangerous and criminal streets because I knew myself to be perfectly safe. I lived in the street and the street looks after its own.

To an outsider, London is all pace and variety. It is such a melting-pot for gay men who are unafraid to be themselves, university dropouts posing as Indian Brahmins, thousands of underpaid workers who stay bright despite their awful living conditions and apparently dreary lives. There are thousands of women with illegitimate children; thousands of small-time crooks (I actually saw the bodies after two gangland killings during my first Christmas in London); thousands of vastly talented people in the arts, thousands of coloured people from all over and millions of tourists. I am told that the old London has ceased to exist. The new London is made up of all these multifarious people blended together. The contrast with Melbourne is absolute. Here, there is no norm. Anything goes. I, too, could be who and what I wanted and still belong. There was only one prerequisite — tolerance.

For someone desperately searching for identity or belonging, London is therefore a great opportunity. In the midst of my struggle to survive, I suddenly realized what I wanted most — to survive. Who would have thought, two years earlier, that I would have been living in Islington, working nights as a barmaid and carrying on a grand love affair with a Cambridge lad all at once? The shy, mixed-up, undirected girl who had watched the lights of Melbourne sink beneath the horizon was changing — from someone who thought herself no good for anything worthwhile, to someone who was deciding that she was probably good for quite a lot. Able to survive at least, just as at fifteen, she had survived in the surf, without Watchers.

Such violent transitions are bound to be long and even painful operations. There were often times when I weakened, pleading with the others in the flat to shut up and let me sleep, threatening them with a full-scale *grand mal* if they did not comply. I could never have turned on a fit at will, but believing I would have one would certainly lower my resistance to such an eventuality. At times like that they thought me a bit crazy. London is not the place for sleeping! Queen Victoria also got her own back, more often than I would have liked to admit. Barmaiding was certainly a tiring job — I was often too tired to sleep. I began to forget night doses of pills, or not have time to take the morning doses. There was a lot of T L E, as a result, usually on my nights off from the pub.

Too exhausted from the day's work to eat properly, I might be resting in my room when someone upstairs put on a record. The bass notes come pounding through the ceiling and walls; boom boom di boom. I can't switch that off. The windows of the room are closed to keep out both dust and traffic noises. That means a shorter supply of oxygen. It is also a hot spring. Finally, when it is too late to do anything about it, I find my eyes fixed on the mirror, staring at the reflection of the electric light bulb. Heat, fatigue, stuffiness, hunger, inadequate drugs, the rhythm of the record — how could I resist the final precipitating factor — the light? Many hours I spent in that odd-shaped London room, unaware of time or place, moaning and wrestling with my little devil. At least these severe attacks served as a reminder to look after myself, which I took notice of for a few days, until London diverted my attention again.

Daring and independence reached greater heights — literally. I met an enthusiastic mountaineer and joined a Polytechnic mountaineering club. This climber was a fanatic. He was a born Scout Leader and treated me like a Boy Scout. But ours was the only tent that stayed up in the Cornish winds. Ours was the only tent that stayed warm in the Welsh snow — Peter zipped up the tent door and lit a candle! Ours was the only tent that stayed dry in the Yorkshire wet. And so I climbed mountains. Wastwater to Scafell Pikes in three feet of snow with a bright blue sky above us. Cwm Silyn — the same. Ingleborough in sun and high winds. Cornwall — the same. I gloried in this new-found occupation, quite beyond all dreams of Emancipation from the Dreaded Disability. Moutaineering, along with swimming (at least alone) is one of those pursuits explicitly denied to an epileptic. Of course, it makes perfectly good sense. Any reasonable person will see the logic behind such debarments and approve of them. But I was not prepared to sacrifice my independence to reason.

I learned to carry my pills in an absolutely waterproof container, whenever we were camping, and to carry a bottle of water in case there was nowhere suitable to drink from along the way. Pete provided the camping and climbing gear, and the extra socks.

Pete was the Meet Secretary. Not being conversant with English society societies, I understood that to mean that he arranged the food supplies. We certainly had more beans and eggs than anyone else. What he really did was to plan the details for each expedition. That was a marvellous year. For months at a time I forgot that I was an epileptic. No bracelet, no fuss, and nobody to tell me I must not climb mountains.

But it was irksome not doing the job I like most — selling books. Backroom work was good training but after a few months I was itching to get back on to the shop floor, facing customers. I just don't work as well in a closed, social situation. The boss drew the line at me going into the retail part of the business. Admittedly there had been a fit while I was on duty before — but only once. So I rebelled and decided to go to Europe. Just like that. Before leaving Australia such a decision would have been unthinkable. But something had happened since I crossed the world alone. The ragged owlet had become a sparrow and was now watching the skylarks with a view to launching out and up.

16

Common sense dictated that if I were to go travelling alone in foreign countries for several months, some sort of identification disc might come in handy — just in case. This time, common sense won, so I bought a doggy-tag, had it inscribed with name, drugs and the word 'Epileptic' (which is hopefully recognizable in all Western languages) and hung it around my neck. That done, I took to collecting drugs.

'Please do not ask your doctor to prescribe medicine for your use while travelling' say the notices in the surgery. It was impossible to get three months' supply of drugs for any reason so I had to resort to crooked ways. I would go to the doctor every three weeks instead of four to get a prescription. The harrased, British GP is unlikely to check the last date on which he handed you one of those myriad strips of paper, so it is quite easy for someone with a chronic complaint to amass a huge amount of drugs. I collected three months' supply extra, which lasted me all summer.

It is a pity that we have to be so surreptitious. Surely the doctors (or the Health Service) should realize that it is much better for an epileptic to stay on the same proven drugs than try to get similar ones from doctors in foreign countries? The drug might not be identifiable, and then follows the possibility of withdrawal symptoms. I regret to say that the only retort I get to this apparently reasonable argument is, 'Well, someone like you shouldn't want to go travelling, anyway.'

But why should I not go travelling? Why should I miss out on such a mind-broadening experience? So many people (including my family) seem to expect me to stay at home and lead the most regular, unvaried, boring life possible. They think it should be sufficient for me just to be still alive. For me that is too much of a submission. It is the very submissiveness of the whole picture that other people paint for me that makes me determined to go so far the opposite way that they will be left speechless. Perhaps it is foolhardy for an epileptic to travel alone. But if you honestly do not believe that there will be a *grand mal* during a certain period and if you definitely do not fear the consequences, even if there is one, then the results will be impressive. It is my experience that, with fairly good drug control, the possibility of having a *grand mal* is considerably lessened by a determined and fearless resistance to the whole disorder.

I used up the remaining money in my Australian bank account to buy a Eurail Pass (unlimited rail travel for three months) and allotted myself £20 a week, all-inclusive, in traveller's cheques. The barmaiding money helped out with a new backpack, a sleeping bag and a warm coat as well as walking boots. I crossed the Channel.

Travelling is fabulous. All the people I met, especially in youth hostels, were young (at least in spirit) and idealistic, and everyone had their story. The oldest youth hosteller I ever met was a South African lady of seventy-eight who was enjoying her retirement greatly. She was 'not quite strong enough' to carry a heavy backpack, so she dragged all her belongings around in two shopping trolleys. Some of us, amazed at her intrepid approach to life, asked her why she preferred to stay at a youth hostel.

'Well, dear,' she said, 'it's all I can afford on my pension, you know!' Another seeker after self-determination.

As it happened, the doggy-tag was never needed. It was a great advantage for me, travelling alone, because people are more likely to begin conversation with a single person. So I managed to meet and talk with a huge variety of people from most countries in the world. Also I could sleep when I felt like it. Two hours in the middle of the day would just about make up for a foreshortened night spent in the same room as forty excited German school girls, or four inexhaustible French teenagers, whose chatter was difficult to quell. I played the ogre now and then.

I have never been so singularly happy and unquestionably healthy in my whole life. Days fell into the non-monotonous regularity of planning the programme, climbing up a mountain, eating a staple diet of chocolate-milk-bananas for lunch, followed by a good sleep in the fresh air, and climbing down the mountain again in the late afternoon. The sun followed me all over Scandinavia, Germany and Austria. There was no suggestion of a fit and even *petit mals* were extremely rare — over three months! In this way I conquered all the glorious mountain scenery from Geiranger to the Dolomites.

Lakes, fjords, mountains, valleys, historic towns — I had seen what I wanted to see in Europe and loved it all. It had been an absolutely successful, independent venture. The sort of venture that is common amongst all young people. The sort of venture that is often simply not on for people like me. And now I was ready to work again. But work was not forthcoming. This time there was no question of me being unemployed because of epilepsy. A million other people were also unemployed, most of them born in Britain.

At this point I managed to get myself hopelessly entangled with British red tape. It was, apparently, a monstrous crime that I did not 'sign on' (my Australian upbringing precludes such measures) with the result that every day I expected to be locked up for not being a burden on the taxpayer. The authorities drew the obvious conclusion that during the subsequent three months in which I was job-hunting, I must have been living with an Italian millionaire in Paris, not living carefully off the remains of my savings like a decayed gentlewoman ought. All my papers seemed to be out of order. Then I discovered something else.

In the British welfare state, if you register as an epileptic you can spend the rest of your life doing nothing, having your drugs paid for and permanently drawing Social Security. For some of us I know that is very necessary and a tremendous help. For the great majority of the rest of us it is a terrible and quite unnecessary temptation. I refuse to register because I simply will not be treated as handicapped. I pay for my drugs because I am too proud to sign all those forms which may save me eighty pence a month. If other people consider me as due for the handicapped category, that is their loss; I know whether or not I can work.

During this most confusing time of unemployment I was rejected for treatment by five doctors' surgeries because the address on my card was wrong (I had just moved), put through a top-to-toe inspection by a Casualty Department because it was the only way to get a new supply of pills, found that a vital form called P45 was missing and that I was expected to produce it or be taxed on emergency rates forever, and found that I owed a huge sum of money to the National Health because they could not account for me for over six months.

It was one of those times when the situation cannot get any worse, so it just has to get better. I decided to leave all of the officials to do what they pleased with their red tape and gratefully accepted an invitation to spend Christmas with friends in Norfolk — turkey and chestnut stuffing and everything on the table home-grown or home-bottled except for the pepper and salt.

A good job turned up within a few days — manageress of a university bookshop in Surrey. Again I told the owner that I have epilepsy; again he dismissed it as irrelevant. My qualifications were what mattered. I got the job. We had some very interesting customers; titled people and celebrities in their Rollses and Jaguars, absent-minded professors and their very bright children. One nine-year boy used to lie on the floor and translate Chaucer with a pencil.

I had not had a *grand mal* during the day for fourteen months when I started there. England was doing me a great deal of good, as were the new drug, garoin, and the simple fact of growing older. It was now eleven years since my first *grand mal* and some improvement could be expected. The shop was doing well and after four months I finally found a place to live, sharing a house with a group of airline pilots and stewardesses — a thoroughly different and exciting world. Everything was beautiful and I was quite convinced (again) that I would never have another *grand mal*. I had forgotten what it meant to have a lifelong label, so much so that I was forgetting to look after myself properly.

An epileptic, however well his fits are controlled, must eat and sleep properly as well as taking the drugs without fail. One night, the airline pilots had a party and I had four hours sleep. The next day I rode my bike to work as usual (it was about two and a half miles to the town), then went for a brains-trust session with the boss. By the time I was riding home again it was six o'clock, fatigue had caught up with me, the pills were three hours overdue, I was hungry and the strain of the meeting had been lifted. I found myself in the local cottage hospital wondering whatever had happened. Only the inevitable, after all.

I was badly bruised, having fallen off the bicycle going at my usual breakneck speed. It felt as if someone had cleft my skull with an axe and the injections they gave me to stop the retching were ineffectual. The shock and defeatism wafting up through the haze and semi-consciousness just made me want to lie down and die. There were no bones broken although the one person who witnessed the accident said that the bike and me had crashed straight to the road, myself still sitting upright in the saddle. One of the pilots came and picked me up, shy of the fit and angry at being disturbed at 11 p.m.: he had been trying to get some sleep before an early flight. I was taken home, vague, ill, and miserable — and terribly angry. So my little devil was still around after all.

It must have taken the hospital staff some five hours to discover my name, drugs, address and telephone number.

Barking questions at me was no way to get information from an epileptic in the post–*grand mal* fuzzy stage. This is the one time when a 'Medic Alert' would certainly have been handy; saved the hospital staff a lot of time and testing for what could possibly be the matter with me; saved me the mentally impossible effort of trying to assimilate the questions and even answering them. Without such a 'Medic Alert', the doctors have every right to believe I have had a heart attack, stroke, overdose; or that I am diabetic, drunk — or possibly — epileptic. And believing me to be a public nuisance by trying to harm myself, they have every right to be impatient and bark questions at me.

'What is your name?' I could not remember. 'Where do you live?' I have no idea — could it be London? or Melbourne? 'What is your phone number?' They may as well have asked me the population of Afghanistan. Numbers are the most difficult things of all to recall after a fit. Finally I pointed to my handbag. There again, they would not find the red card of the British Epileptic Association — it would have been useful. But they did find a pillbox with garoin and tegretol in it, so they were finally able to diagnose the probable cause of the fall from the bicycle and the nurses were instantly kinder to me. I was grateful — but also cross that a hospital might presume alcohol or drugs before thinking of diabetes or epilepsy.

That fit was a bitter disappointment. Worse than all the bruises and the mangled state of my precious bicycle was that it set me right back psychologically. I was once more afraid of people and avoided parties or any sort of challenge. The best way of curing that attitude was, I knew, to become a barmaid again. In a pub I could meet a lot of people without the necessity of much actual involvement in their private lives. I went to a local posh pub and worked behind the bar in my Indian clothes and headband. The local millionaires excused me, again, on the grounds of coming from 'down under'; so we enjoyed solving the world's problems together over a ginger beer.

Barmaiding, I knew from experience, also had its dangers.

Fatigue and an irregular life were leading to frequent bouts of T L E again. By this time I knew what to call them, and, within a few hours after one extensive session, I decided to write down what I could remember about it, piecing the process together from the conscious bits and trying to guess what happened in between. Here is the result.

I'm tired from a social occasion the night before. Terribly hungry because I missed breakfast so as to get to work in time, missed morning coffee to make up for lateness — my lunch-hour is at two. So is pill-time and it is nearly that now. It's a busy, three-hour session on the shop floor with people firing unceasing questions at me. Normally I thrive on being busy but today it's too much. Somebody asks about a book . . . (switch off half-way, so I don't know what they want) . . . question must be answered. He's standing there waiting for me (fumbling in catalogues and drawers to gain time). He looks impatient so that can't be right. I feel stifled; I can't speak. There's a drill boring into the middle of my forehead, churning up the thought processes. I can't hear. There's a high-pitched note ringing in my ears (Somebody says I better go to lunch because I look tired.) Cross the street, Press the lift button. Little things like lift-buttons can become totally absorbing at times like this. Can't find my way to the restaurant. (Walk uncertainly around the various departments, looking for all the world like a very green shop-lifter.) In the restaurant I stand and look vaguely around. What am I doing here? Where am I? (Sit down, get up again, sit down somewhere else. Look miserably, helplessly at people, unrecognizing.) The waitresses are of the old, white shirt and black skirted school.

"Your usual, madam?" (I can't answer. Don't understand the question — just know it must be answered.) "Take your time, madam."

Later, "Are you sure you're all right, madam?" (Terribly hot in here, can't pour the tea, forget my 'sloppy eggs on toast' are waiting. I just get up and go, without paying. Hope the oxygen outside will help.)

But the intensely cold wind on my forehead only seems

to make a game of it. I can feel my temples humming — not really a pain but an inescapable feeling. I'm near to tears and gasping with frustration. The shopping list is useless because I can't reason where to go. It's like a jammed electric system buzzing away in my head and I can't unjam it. I roam aimlessly through the market stalls, pick things up, try to buy something I want but don't know whether I've already asked for it or only imagined that I have — the stall-holder is looking suspiciously at me so I pay. Forget to take the item (don't know what it is, return to ask price again and pay again). Must go to the bank. What for? (Teller would like to know also.) It's a hopeless situation so I rush back to work, more by instinct than design.

All afternoon it continues. I get shaky. Rush up and down, not knowing what I want. Desperately want to cry but can't. Give double directions to staff. "Are you all right?" asks one lady, puzzled at the way I keep staring at her. I don't answer — I don't know the answer. Spend three times as long as usual over a short letter. I am frustrated to screaming point in my attempts to throw the thing off. In moments of consciousness I know it's happening but there's no way I can swim up to the top and get out of the drowning, rushing torrent of continual brainstorms misfiring.

During T L E, I always want to scream loudly, but never do. No amount of breathers or coffees will stop it — only a good rest uninterrupted by the necessity to take part in conversations, or carry on any important work. As with *grand mal*, it takes much longer to realize that I am indeed in such a state if I am alone, than if I have a sympathetic friend nearby who can make me lie down, turn off the light or whatever may have been the final causal factor and simply wait silently until it all goes away.

T L E is genuinely dangerous. It always seems to result from a conglomeration of factors — heat, fatigue, hunger, nearness to pill-time, hectic social intercourse in which certain things are expected of me in some capacity. Most of those could have been eliminated by my own foresight each time. Further factors like flickering lights and piercing sounds must be avoided by practice, because there are only a few moment's grace before it will be too late to avoid them. I sometimes wonder what would happen if the scream just inside my throat ever really surfaced. Obviously, all my normal faculties of sight, smell, speech, hearing, understanding and basic reasoning are variously just not present, or else are intensified to blot out all the other senses, over a period of several hours. Perhaps I really have nine lives or a guardian angel because something outside myself has so far prevented me from being run over when crossing busy roads in a trance, or falling over the side of a ship or a cliff for that matter

T L E attacks have usually followed some extra stress. But I can find no rule to help prevent them. I never think about such things while in examinations, which for most people are full of stress; or while mountaineering, which at least puts people on their mettle; or while swimming or doing anything which I enjoy. T L E seems to have developed in me as *grand mal* has become less frequent. Epilepsy goes in cycles — I may have no *grand mal* for two years, and then have seven or eight in six months. It is hard not to regress to an unhappy dependence during the latter periods; hard not to get things out of proportion, again.

While working at my new pub job I began to go out with a Scot who was pleasant enough — except that he found it absolutely necessary to consume ten pints a day. Not of carrot juice. He found it difficult to communicate until he was at least half-way through his quota — and after that he was not really worth communicating with. So I met a Welsh boat-builder from Dartmouth and fell in love with him instead. We met initially because he came into the bookshop inquiring after a paperback entitled *Been Down For So Long It Looks Like Up to Me*, which was mercifully out of print. After that we started meeting in the local park and finally he went back to Dartmouth where I spent an enchanting holiday.

Unfortunately, I still had the weakness to tell boy-friends straight away that I am an epileptic. Perhaps it was a sort of defence, but the outcome really depends on our reasons for telling people, the way we told them and in what context. I was still doing it for the wrong reasons in the wrong way and at the wrong time. This was unfortunate because however liberal-minded they were it could not help but make a difference in their attitudes towards me. Sometimes they assigned ordinary individuality to epileptic causes or made too many allowances. Knowledge of the presence of such a factor as epilepsy can make a partner very considerate, but it can also put up a wall so that he knows that he does not want to get totally involved. Now I would prefer to be known and cared about as a person first, letting the discovery of the extra factor come across naturally, much later. There is the reasonable and valid argument that says — What if you have a *grand mal* in front of him without having told him? I think it is worth taking the risk. I may only go out with someone a few times, just to see how well we get on. Why bring in any complicating factor so early? That way I may never know the man's true feelings. Why even bother to think about it? It may cloud the enjoyment of the outing. But if he is the One and Only, when you do tell him, it only adds respect to love. Never mind. It was all good experience for me — the sort of experience I should have had six or eight years earlier.

One day I was stuck at home with a cold and nothing to read. The bookshelves of my friends, the airline pilots, were packed full of Flight Manuals, true air adventure stories, air force war stories, imagined aeroplane situation adventure stories — and one other book, *The Devil Rides Out*, by Dennis Wheatley. I read it from cover to cover in one lying, my horror increasing at each page, not at the witchcraft so much as at the author's ignorant, uninformed usage of the term 'epileptic'. I was, by that time, emancipated enough about my disorder to see red when it is described in a way that can only make the reading public set us apart as something to be either avoided or ridiculed. No wonder people can be frightened or horrified when they discover that they or their children have epilepsy! No wonder they would have wished anything else upon them than that! My indignation reached its height on reading this occult, black mass thriller. It sowed such a seed of wrath that within a year the first draft of this book had been written.

An impartial reader with no immediate knowledge of epilepsy could easily conclude from some of Wheatley's descriptions that epileptics are abnormal and unbalanced, that they are frustrated in every way because of their disability and find some compensation in being able to side with the devil in such rituals. If the reader were soon to be introduced to a real epileptic he could be excused for not wanting anything to do with him.

In the same book, during a satanic attack on one man in a group the man starts 'shaking like an epileptic in a fit'. Frankly, I do not think this likeness is necessary or even appropriate. Let the man shake if he must — but why liken him to an epileptic? To the vast majority of people it would be more meaningful if he was likened to a dog having a nightmare, something which most people have at least seen. The original, unfair likeness presumes a connection between epilepsy and satanic possession. Surely not even the most superstitious and fearful layman could possible make such a connection in the civilized world? But for people who are just reading the book for entertainment and who may glean such damaging non-information in passing, seeing these statements in black and white can only give a shock of doubt.

When my cold was bearable and I had returned to work, I purposely set out to read Dostoevsky's *The Idiot* again, as an antidote to the appalling injustice of the satanic black mass. This time it had a wonderful, warming, familiar effect on me. I read it without a trace of the defiances and defences of eight years before, basking instead in the tremendous perception and illumination of the author.

At last I was ready for such an experience.

Life for me is one long series of great ups and enormous
downs followed inevitably by an even greater up than before. It is like surfing or flying. Perilous, exhilarating —
a fulltime experience. I fall, but on my feet. So, in the midst
of coping well with this small management job, being in
love, working nights as a barmaid and having a stable, happy
place to live, it was only a matter of time before something
went wrong. This time it was the Home Office.

My annual visa was due for renewal. No problems,
thought I, just take a good book and a picnic lunch to the
Home Office and wait in the line — there are usually about
600 people queueing there at any one time. But there
were problems. I was declared an alien and given eight days
to leave the country. No Work Permit? Not engaged in
full-time study? Not married to someone in the above
categories? Then — out. But my employer says I am in-
dispensable and irreplaceable! Sorry. But my grandfather
was born here! Prove it — in eight days.

I was in a great state of shock. The people, and especially
the pavement, which had looked so friendly on the way
to the Home Office had become instantly foreign on the
way back. Everything looked hostile. Although I am a
sixth-generation Australian on most sides, my ancestors
all came from Britain at one time. But now I was just an
outsider with eight days left.

I did not want to go home. I was not ready to go home.
A premature return might mean a regression to my former
state of unhappy, insecure, self-preoccupation and dependence. The good lady from the Home Office would not
even allow a short extension to give me time to find the
birth certificate of my grandfather, who was killed at
Ypres in 1917. There was a major obstacle to this. Nobody
knew where he was born and there were at least fifty
Walter Scotts born in the same quarter as him. Besides,
when I admitted that his name was Walter Scott, it made

the whole affair even less believable.

Finally, I took a chance. I went back to the Home Office with only three days to go and began my story at the other end, the search for my grandfather. As a result I was given a year to find Walter, provided I did not work. But the shock of having the earth taken out from under me so suddenly was undiminished. I ran away to Wales. The boat-builder I found in Surrey had a friend there whose caravan was vacant and needed minding. I moved in, with one pack full of belongings on my back. There was neither electricity nor sanitation and winter was coming. I did not even have a transistor radio. With that unpromising start, the search for the real Walter Scott began.

17

Time passes. Try Manchester — no luck. Try Sheffield
— no luck. War Graves Commission — no information.
Desperation sets in. Shock of alienation unabated. Re-
moteness of dwelling does not help. But the dog does,
though.

She was the last of a litter of pups from a stray bitch
taken in by the local fruit and vegetable merchant. I had
never realized how very intelligent and lovable these shaggy,
black and white sheepdogs can be. Nobody wanted Kate
because one of the fruit and vegetable man's five little
daughters had accidentally poured boiling water on her
when she was a tiny bundle of a puppy. There was a ugly
scar from the base of her head to the middle of her back.
But I wanted her, passionately. I needed her. So we each
did the other a good turn by adopting one another. As I
carried her home through the mist, I talked softly all the
way, telling her her name and where she was going to live
and how badly I wanted a friend right then. She has never
left my side since. Faithful little hound — problems were
never so big once I had Kate and Kate had me. Moreover,
she gave me a good excuse for talking to myself again.

We spent the whole winter in that caravan on a moun-
tainside in Wales. There was not a tremendous amount
of snow, but there were frequent frosts. It was also the year
of the January hurricane which, miraculously, did not over-
turn our extremely exposed dwelling, although it brought
down dozens of huge beech trees on the farm. It was an
old 'Bluebird' —type caravan with a little gypsy stove which,
an hour or two after being lit, made the caravan so warm
that the butter melted and I would sit in a shimmy with
the frosts biting harmlessly at the draughty windows.

Coming from Australia. I had never really understood the term 'frozen stiff' until I awoke one morning to find the snowdrops frozen into their vase, some washing which had been left soaking frozen into the sink, the water carrier full of useless, immovable ice, and, most curious, the chemical toilet transformed into an iceberg two feet high!

If ever I was to learn total independence, there was no better way than living in such a wild, remote place with so few resources — and over a winter into the bargain. The nearest shop was five miles away. The short days were all taken up with carting, drying and chopping wood, fetching water or walking — elementary survival. The long nights had to be passed somehow. I soon indulged in the luxury of a transistor radio; Kate was wonderful to talk to, but I needed something to talk back at me occasionally. The interminable night-times became sessions of sewing, knitting toys for the farm children, doing tapestry, darning socks and becoming thoroughly acquainted with the B B C.

It was during this time of intensive listening that I heard a modern radio play which made me nearly as angry as the black mass thrillers. It was depicting the problems of convicted sex offenders at the mercy of fellow prisoners. Suddenly, for no significant reason, one man was represented as a serious epileptic and sex offender in the same speech. His fellow prisoners were extremely cruel to him, nearly drowning him in the bath. Intensive surveys show no connection whatsoever between any sort of crime and epilepsy. Between all of us, we will show the entire spectrum of possible morality, from saintliness to evil, just as in society as a whole. I fail to see the necessity for such a dubious connection in this play unless it had been followed up and presented directly with a special object in mind.

On the other hand, the B B C 'Waggoner's Walk', has as a principal character an epileptic. She is a young girl whose boyfriend knows about the problem and has decided that it is not central to their relationship. She is represented as a normal, happy, young woman who happens to have *grand mal* at about the same rate as me. The difficulties she encounters trying to get a job in her chosen profession and her reaction to these setbacks are no better and no worse than I know them to be, and I am grateful that so many people all over Britain will become familiar with this character. It can only educate for good.

In searching the library for facts to counter the suppositions in the first-mentioned play, I came across an amazing statement, written only two years previously. An author was surmising about the medical history of famous people in previous centuries, from accounts written by people who knew them. One of the chosen characters was Napoleon Bonaparte, who is often supposed to have been an epileptic. In describing Napoleon's fits of anger, the writer goes on

. . . these attacks, observed by untrained witnesses, have given rise to the statment that Napoleon was the subject of epilepsy . . . . Bursts of passion and severe vomiting followed by lethargy are poor facts on which to *brand a man with the stigma of epilepsy . . .* ' (My italics).

CHAPLIN, *Tenements of Clay*, 1974.

Can this really show the attitude of an apparently medical man to epilepsy — in 1974?

The old Bluebird was sited in a corn field, on a hill above the farmhouse, and about half a mile away. We had a magnificent view of the Prescellies. Every day I hoped to find some proof of my British origins, which would allow me to stay and work without reapplying for a visa. My mother was working wonders with her business letters in Australia but there seemed no hope of finding old Walter's birthplace. He emigrated at the age of twenty-two and was killed at twenty-seven. Meanwhile the cycle of fits was once more in its darkest quarter. I should not have been upset about the dramatic increase in *grand mals* — but it just did not make the overall picture of life at that time look any brighter. I had at least four serious *grand mals* over six months, not counting night fits.

After the first one, I tottered down to the farmhouse in a bewildered, unhappy way. The lady was very kind, but as I could not answer her questions as to what had happened she was rather alarmed. At least I could shake my head when she suggested getting a doctor. But the death-fear was overwhelming in me and I whimpered like a puppy for some time. Kate was tightly clasped in my arms, herself only eight weeks old. Eventually her wriggling diverted me enough to laugh and I was finally able to accept a cup of tea and explain briefly what the matter was. The lady of the house was terribly upset.

'What!' she exlaimed. 'You shouldn't be living up there, all alone. Anything might happen!' She was right of course, in her way, but instinctively I knew that I was right, too.

It had been quite a bad *grand mal*. I was covered with bruises having banged my head and arms all over the small kitchen area. It was a great disappointment and it seemed to me that my propensity for having fits was getting worse. But I need not have worried. The large gap between *grand mals* only served to make me forget what they felt like. So when they did come, it was a much greater shock to the system than when I used to have two dozen or so every year. It took that much longer to realize what had happened, and that much longer to rationalize the death-fear.

During the ensuing few days when I was in the usual, frail state, I spoke quite a lot to the family about epilepsy. They were very interested and concerned. It was a weakness, this not being able to help putting myself under the protection of people who had seen me during, or shortly after a *grand mal*. I needed to play the helpless role and it invariably altered our relationship. I felt vulnerable and inadequate with such people. just as anyone feels uneasy when in the presence of somebody who knows their character weakness. A gambler with his creditors. An easy woman with a nun. A small-time crook with a probation officer. A husband who hides his dirty socks from his spotless wife. That is how I felt.

The next *grand mal* was much worse. It was during
Christmas when all the neighbours for a mile around were
away. There are two days which are almost wiped clean
in my memory, except for the occasional moments of
consciousness. It is probable that I had two or three *grand
mals* in succession. I can remember the headache and
crawling along the caravan floor to get water from the
container. Goodness know how long that took! Making a
pot of tea is an automatic reaction for me so that was not
so difficult. It is absolutely necessary to have pills after a
fit, as soon as my stomach can keep them down. Well,
I kept trying. Providence had decreed a warmish Christmas which was merciful because I had no fire over those
two days. Each time I awoke I would find myself on the
floor, or perhaps half-propped on one of the built-in
caravan seats with little Kate licking my face earnestly,
in a worried sort of way, and finally in a hungry sort of
way. It was she who eventually forced me to rouse myself
properly in order to make her some warm, puppy-food.
At last I could smile at her eagerness. But the death-fear
had been terrible. I hope, fervently, that I never have
such a prolonged succession of *grand mals* again. With Kate
alternately nuzzling my face and sitting up straight in a
perplexed way. I could hear myself moaning and then
crying, begging her not to die either. She was already the
single most important being in my life.

On the third day, the fear was dissipated and we went
for a long walk in the pouring rain, marvelling at the most
intricate patterns which rain made down the bark of trees.
Also, I taught Kate to 'fetch'. She brought me her bright,
orange, rubber lion, laid it at my feet and wagged her tail
hopefully, peering up at me from the great height of
twelve inches. The terrifying aftermath of a *grand mal*
always goes completely away, but I can not seem to remember that when it is happening.

It was made worse, this bad part of the cycle, by the
loneliness. My boat-builder had returned to Dartmouth,
his sister had gone away and I knew not a soul, except the

farmer's family, within two hundred miles. Of necessity I made a few friends; most lived at least an hour's walk away and all were busy with their own lives. My life seemed to be in suspension although it was, admittedly, full of fresh air, surrounded by breathtaking scenery (or thick fog, or a solid sheet of rain) and it embraced a dream, living alone in the wilderness, which many people would love to realize but never get the opportunity.

This constant aloneness was pretty harrowing at first, but it turned out to be another blessing in disguise. I was not very successful at living with other people. What better place to learn how to live on my own? When you are left solely in the company of yourself for a long time, you had better make the best of it, or you might not come out the other end. So, with Kate's help, I did. I filled every minute and came to learn a whole lot more about survival and my own resources. The words of *Desiderata*, 'Many fears are born of fatigue and loneliness', applied even more strongly to me now. During that difficult yet salutary first six months in my Welsh wilderness, I learned how to combat the paranoia and the feeling that life was getting at me somehow by the simple expedient of counting my blessings. I would begin with being alive, having a pot of hot tea and seeing the sun shining; then I could progress to − at least the dog loves me, which led to how many friends wrote me letters last week, and so on, till the whole framework of the temporary lapse in spirit would disintegrate.

I became very fit in Wales. Up where we lived, there were definitely no buses so I had to find another method of getting to the bank (to withdraw from my rapidly depleted savings again) and then to the shops, to buy anything that was 'on special'. Farmers are very busy people. A few times I got lifts with them into the town but it was useless making a permanent arrangement. It was seventeen miles to the market town − too far even for someone like John

Hillaby to walk there and back, carrying a pack loaded with a week's shopping one way. I was naturally ineligible for a driving licence.

People who have cars or friends with cars simply cannot understand the problems of someone who is desperate to get somewhere and can't drive. With public transport so hideously expensive (not to mention shrinking if not non-existent), there is really only one solution -- shanks pony and hitch. To this argument I get a similar answer to my views on travelling: 'If you can't drive and can't afford a chauffeur then you should not live alone and, what is more, you should not want to go anywhere. You should just accept the situation.'

I should just accept it -- or make someone else's life a misery by living with them and asking them to drive me around. Not likely. Before we bought Harriett at college, I used to hitch-hike as a student, but everyone expects students and people in the forces to hitch. Now I was ten years older. Having Harriett was all very well at the time, because we were living in a close community. But it would be no use me buying a car if it might take me a week to find someone even to drive me into the village. So I walked and hopefully stuck out my thumb.

Here enters Queen Victoria again, closely followed by a nonchalent, determined Barbra Streisand.

QV: Now dear -- I really can't allow you to go . . . er . . . hitchhiking.
BS: Why not? Lots of people do it.
V: Quite plainly it indicates a lack of moral fibre. It is tantamount to begging.
B: Rubbish. I have to work hard for a lift. Drivers expect to be entertained.
V: (shocked) What *do* you mean? It is extremely dangerous. There is entertainment and er . . . entertainment.
B: Oh really! You make it sound as if all drivers are potential sex maniacs . . .
V: It only takes one, dear. Moreover, you are too old for

such capers.

B: Not at all! Life is just beginning. My face doesn't matter. It simply needs a certain sort of happy, self-confidence.

V: You can do just as well with public transport — if you really must go somewhere.

B: What? On my bank account! Oh — hitch-hiking gives me much more freedom.

V: Yes, freedom to be murdered.

B: Over Kate's dead body.

After the first few times, when my thumb trembled so much and my face was so tense that it is a wonder that the drivers did not report me to the police as a suspicious character, Kate and I became quite adept at hitch-hiking. She got me a lot of lifts. When we climbed into the car people would say, 'I don't usually pick up hitch-hikers — but I saw the dog.' She still gets lifts for me, sitting up straight beside my backpack with a clean, white shirt-front, and looking reproachfully at everyone who passes us. If I fall asleep on my feet (my thumb still out), she lets me know that someone has stopped by rushing towards the car, just to make sure, then rushing back to me again with an excited bark.

Not being allowed to drive is the greatest threat to a controlled epileptic's independence. Once, in desperation, after trying to get to the doctor for a new supply of pills, I did indeed write a big notice saying, 'Trying to get to the doctor.' It was a busy enough road and a handy place to stop. Kate and I stood there for a total of three and a half hours, then crossed the road and hitched home again, without the necessary prescription. There have been plenty of times like that. But generally, I adore hitching — so does Kate.

When I first arrived in Wales, I had one pack of belongings and a sleeping bag. All the other stuff was left in Surrey. So we hitched down with an empty pack, once a week, then back again with it full. Up and down the famous M4. It was a marvellous experience. I would take a thermos and have tea and sandwiches in the middle of some swirling roundabout, not envying the drivers. Moreover, you can see so much more of the countryside from the passenger seat — especially in a transcontinental lorry. When I got really fed up with being alone and knew that I was getting things out of proportion, Kate and I would do a marathon, twelve-hour hitch to Cambridge where we stayed with the rare sort of friends that do not mind people dropping on them out of the blue, ate Sunday dinners with chocolate cake, wore a skirt for a change and went window-shopping. Then we could return to Wales knowing that everything was all right, really.

If an epileptic is having *grand mal* as frequently as I am, then he will know that he may never drive. Not everyone may take the alternative of hitch-hiking, but it is imperative that we come to terms with this early on and find our own solution to the problem of getting ourselves around without bothering other people too much. It is just possible for a controlled epileptic to get permission to drive a motor vehicle. The law requires a medical tribunal to find that there have been no fits for three years. In fact, I can drive a car. There are plenty of deserted roads in the Australian outback. As with surfing, I never felt more alert and competent than when I was driving. But my family were too horrified at the possibility that I might kill someone else as well as myself. I know they are right. Some years ago there was a case in Melbourne of a woman who had an epileptic fit at the wheel of her car, causing a head-on collision. She was slightly hurt. Three other people were killed. The judge let her go free on the grounds that she was not conscious at the time. But how to bear such guilt for the rest of one's life? I do not drive.

Hitch-hiking has taught me much about drivers in general and it is just fortunate that I am not a nervous passenger. After hitching some 40,000 miles, I consider that I would be far less dangerous than at least half the people on the roads; those who drink three double whiskies or six pints, those who are easily irritated with other drivers and im-

175

patient, not to mention accustomed to getting their own way; those who learned to drive before the war and are not going to change now; those who are subject to heart attacks, headaches or even violent allergies. Surely I would be a safer driver than people with children crying and fighting in the back seat; or with chihuahuas snapping at their earrings, or beating time to their cassette music on the accelerator and brakes, putting on makeup, having a shave, sitting cheek-to-cheek, reading newspapers and consulting maps over the steering-wheel or even filling a pipe — is anybody safe? But there are thousands of excellent drivers as well. It is lucky that I enjoy hitch-hiking. In spite of being an epileptic and having no means of transport, like the singer, 'I've been everywhere, man . . . .'

It was strange, on reflection, how completely I accepted my way of life in that caravan. I doubt that this acceptance was due to a new resilience; probably it was more owing to a sort of shock, make worse by the bad cycle of *grand mals*. In a lonely, vulnerable, bewildered state of mind, my discrimination was apt to be poor. Sometimes people who frequently gave me lifts invited me home, thus I met and got to know one young man who taught me quite a lot. Firstly, he was amazed at the patience I showed in waiting for the authorities to do something about my grandfather. He offered to pay me for cleaning his absolutely filthy bachelor's quarters. I took that on willingly enough although it was a thankless task. Each week I would return to find it in an equally disgusting state. He washed no dishes between my visits and let everything lie where it fell, knowing that I would pick it up. Secondly we became good friends, mainly through our dogs, and he gave me several excellent hints on how to raise a puppy at a very opportune time. Finally he offered me 'dope'. I have never bothered with tobacco and had no idea how to smoke a cigarette. Only once did I try to smoke this home-rolled joint. The effect was so immediate and forceful that after a few draws the Terror came upon me to an alarming degree. The drill in my forehead was almost tangible and I was terrified. 'Dope' is not for epileptics. The chemical combination of our drugs and marihuana must be formidable.

Since that terrible, indescribable experience I have been able to come to a happy conclusion about all the drug-taking necessary for an epileptic. We certainly are free of ever needing to become addicted to any of today's social drugs. We don't even need alcohol or cigarettes to give us an 'up' or a 'trip'. We can get high — on life. We already experience the intensity of vision, hearing and understanding which many people try to get through illegal drug-taking. In *The Idiot*, Mishkin even likens the visions of Mahommed to the 'beatific moments' of an epileptic. I know what he means — what a privilege!

When I told that particular young man about my epilepsy there was very little reaction and I was not hoping for one. I simply told him what happened when I smoked his dope and why I was not going to smoke any more. He in turn agreed that it was probably better not to smoke anything. Because I had not appealed to his sympathy and protection, I did not receive any.

The great majority of people with whom we come in daily contact will never see us in a fit. With them I believe that it is much better not to confide the fact of our epilepsy, unless we're absolutely sure of our personal reasons for this confidence — and that the reasons are definitely not in the 'I'm-an-epileptic-so-you've-got-to-be-nice-to-me' category. It might give us a few advantages but it takes away a whole lot more that are worth the risk.

If we want to be equal with the rest of the world (or at least start out as equal) then we must claim only the basic, common, human problems and traits. It is the only way to find out what sort of a person we are. Some epileptics take advantage of their situation by throwing fits at will which could appear to be genuine, but are simply temper-tantrums. They are not helping the rest of us. If I did that (and I don't think that I could as it is the exact opposite to my whole philosophy) I would deserve a bucket of cold water and a kick in the behind — and hopefully I would still have a friend left to administer said treatment.

That Welshman's singular lack of interest in what had once been my great secret was a reflection of the way I had told him, as well as a reflection of his own liberality of thought. Like the people on the ship, it was as easy for him to accept epilepsy as it was to accept brown hair or large feet. The farmer's concern and worry that I should be living alone is a much more common reaction. If ever I find myself in a position which requires such a confidence, I find that the vast majority of people express a similar concern; their first words are 'Oh, dear! What do I do if you have a fit right now?' I always tell them that it is extremely unlikely, but if it should happen, please — leave me alone to come out of it. And that is usually the end of the subject. Medical histories, however involved or unusual, always become boring, so with the 'concerned' category of people, also, I am able to continue a conversation just as if they had been inquiring politely whether I have had enough lunch, dear.

Doing a lot of hitch-hiking, I often became so exasperated by the drivers' continual insinuations that I should have a job, a car, and a husband rather than thumbing around Britain, that I told them first about the problem with the Home Office (to which the universal reaction was anger against the authorities) and then, if they persisted about the driving, I would explain that I was not allowed to drive. It intrigued me that there was a similar response to that which I had experienced during the university years: 'Oh really? Well that explains everything.' I still get rather frustrated trying to work out that 'everything' is. My way of life? My attitudes? My opinions? Then I get just a little bit sad that there is still so much needing explanation. I never wanted to be very different, after all.

A more formidable repercussion which is noticeable in some city people is that they tend to cancel any public engagement which they may have with me for fear that I should have a fit and embarrass them in front of other friends. These people tell me slowly but firmly the reason for such cancellations. It is understandable on their part and inexcusable on my part for telling them in the first place. True independence is not telling people that I am an epileptic. Not because I want to keep it a secret, but because I want to be judged and included on my own, individual personality. Epilepsy need only be a very small part of my personality — if I want it that way — and its importance in my life can be automatically diminished, at will.

Then there have been the serious, open-minded types. On speaking to a proposed landlady in Cambridge I disclosed the disability for obvious reasons. We had a discussion with her husband. 'Come on,' she said, 'You'd better put all your cards on the table and tell him straight away. You're an epileptic, aren't you?'

It sounds like making a confession. Again, largely my own fault for the way I explained it to them. As it turned out these people had had a previous experience with a particularly unpleasant child who had also been an epileptic. Not all of us are saints like Mishkin — we will show the whole cross-section of human nature. But whereas folks usually take other people as they come, I have found that they tend to bunch us all at one end of the spectrum, depending on their past experience. That is another good reason for not telling people — they will not have to dig into all their preconceptions by which to judge us.

18

Six months after going into retreat there still seemed no hope of being able to work legally again. Money was getting very low and I was desperate enough to do anything just to free myself until something definite happened. So I took on a cash job as a petrol-pump attendant, early in spring, at 40p an hour. It was bitterly cold, going out on to the forecourt to fill-er-up. I wore a bright red, woollen cap with a bobble on the end and an old parka. When I forgot my mittens it was miserable. Being out of season there were not many cars, so I took Kate and the transistor radio. One freezing day I was in the middle of a very exciting play when someone pulled up in an old Rover. Unwilling to part from my play, I took the tranny outside (held close to my ear), and went through the usual procedures — oil, water, tyres and petrol. The driver was furious. He got out in the blasting, icy wind and literally shook his fist at me.

'Listen here young lad,' he began.

'I'm a lady.' I retorted. That set him back a bit.

'Well, young woman,' he continued.

'I'm a lady', I repeated.

'Listen, you', he yelled. 'It's people like you who are destroying the moral tone of this country. Someone should take you in hand. You should be in the army — that'd change your ideas.' (He was still apparently convinced that I was a lad.) I bet it would, thought I, and grinned widely.

'Standing there, more interested in your stupid music, so-called music, than in serving your customers.' He went on, and finally lunged at the radio. I was filling his petrol tank by then. I held on to the tranny but he got petrol all down his impeccable trousers. I put on my best Oxford accent and said, 'This happens to be a very important radio play on Radio 4. Please stop interrupting me.' So that job was finished. I was tired of being called 'lad' and 'boy' all the time. Welsh girls are still expected to wear skirts.

Then came a telegram: 'Australian Army records show Walter Scott born Pontefract Yorkshire love Mum.' Hurray, hurray! I raced down to the new equivalent of Somerset House, and it took only five minutes to find old Walter (or young Walter, as he was when he was born) and two days to procure the full certificate. I was legal!

The fight was over; the pressure was off and, inevitably, I had another *grand mal*. But this time, this time it just did not seem so bad. Kate was also getting used to the phenomenon and would wait, staring at me with great interest, paws stretched out in front. I could even feel her tail thumping on the caravan floor as I regained consciousness. That *grand mal* just could not dampen my high spirits. I determined to go and visit the University College Hospital specialist again. It was from him that I learned about cycles; I was not to worry — it would definitely improve again. All niggling thoughts and halfbaked suspicions about serious brain deterioration were set aside, and I felt a new enthusiasm for life. Spring was coming. Kate was less dispensable, more adorable each day and I was legal again. Being unhappy with the obligatory position that a free caravan put me in, I moved to another one — larger, airier, more beautifully positoned than I could have dreamed. A place to get absolutely well again, to throttle my little devil for ever.

With the spring came the end of the intensive cycle of *grand mals*. Our new home looked over a peaceful and forgotten Welsh valley. I had to walk three miles, even to get to a road with cars on it. Kate did not mind but I wore out quite a few pairs of shoes on that track. I also became very familiar with the abundance of wild flowers, which were a constant joy. As spring turned to the hottest summer on record for many years in Britain, things began to sort themselves out in my mind. I had certainly survived those six wintry, lonely months, dark in every way — but now they no longer appeared to have been so dark. That time had been very similar to my experience with the burns — a spectacular trial from which I had managed to emerge with a new look at life. A period of intensive learning.

Wales is beautiful. But there is no need to sing her praises. She is the last bastion of solitude for eccentrics. She fairly bristles with them. For me there was romance in the all-enveloping mists, the endless rain and the bare thorn bushes. There was unexpected exhilaration in tramping for miles in the freezing wind just to visit a friend who probably wasn't in and take the dog for some fresh air. And there was ecstasy in all the happenings of spring. The possibilities glowed, flared up and grew into a radiant sun. I sat back and basked in this new way of life.

The local farmers, though friendly enough, had already decided that I was a bit strange. I was not married with seven children and a home. I did not have a steady job with an annual holiday on the Costa del Sol, I did not appear to require many possessions, and I was a hitch-hiker. I didn't mind. They could take me as they found me. But they were never to know how very much I had become conscious of over the previous six months; how tremendous it was for me to begin formulating my own, well-proven, elementary rules for epileptics living in the normal adult world.

Most importantly, there is a certain amount of self-control involved in epilepsy. I believe that a good number of fits can be avoided by simply not expecting them. The little devil does not enjoy being ignored — he goes away and sulks. Fits can also be avoided by eating regularly (little and often: I find it an excellent excuse to have a bar of chocolate or an ice-cream); by sleeping well (this need not conflict with a happy social life — it just means being careful); by avoiding all everyday drugs, from aspirin to alcohol, unless absolutely necessary; and by never, never missing the essential pills. It helps to remember, and it is easy to forget even after so many years, if pills are included in a ritual. Being a tea addict helps because whenever I have a pot of tea it follows automatically that I must have a dose of pills. They are, incidentally, kept in the tea caddy! At the time of writing, I have five pill-times per day. Three are accompanied by tea and two are taken with weak coffee. I do not allow pill-time to be an onerous task; it is always a pleasure.

I never avoid going out just because I might not have an opportunity to take them. I have a large handbag containing a water bottle and my latest pillbox, a present from Liz. There are enough doses in it to tide me over until the next day — the last thing I want is to have to decline an overnight invitation. But there have been pill predicaments, several times. In each case I have gone to the nearest casualty department and explained that I had left my pills at home. Better that than interrupt an interesting social situation. One Christmas I was stuck in Norfolk with a whole bottle of tegretol — but not a single garoin tablet in its foil jacket. I went to the Norwich General Hospital. The only other outpatient was a lady who had broken her wrist while dancing on Christmas Eve. The nurses in casualty were extremely kind.

'Oh, we get lots of people like you at Christmas,' they said.

It helps if you can learn to laugh about the *grand mals*. One morning, during that glorious, almost Australian summer, the lady who owned my caravan came to give me my mail. As a surprise, she also brought a bright purple petunia in a little pot. The colour must have been too much for me as it is the last thing that I remember until several hours later. This person had never seen anyone in a fit before, but she later described the usual progress, as always reported, plus the fact of me walking up and down the field, going purposelessly from one row of beans to another, dressed in a very skimpy night dress. All her pleas to put a dressing-gown on, for the Welsh morning was cold, were met by bland uncomprehending stares. Despite the lady's alarm at the sight of a *grand mal*, and my own shrinking from the imagination of what she had seen, we were both able to laugh at the memory of the Maiden amongst the Bean-Stalks.

Another elementary rule that I learned soon after this *grand mal:* I must not expect life to be all sunshine and dandelions. Whose life is? There are times of depression and regression; the important thing being that I now know they will end. Liz arrived during one of these bad times. I had finally persuaded this confirmed Australophile to come and see what she was not missing, if only to be certain that she was not missing anything. It was good to see her again — we had not met for eight years. I wanted to show her Kate and Wales and my way of life. But I was too miserable.

'I'll never get properly well,' I moaned. 'I still have fits — too many — and I still don't like people very much. I'm still no good to anybody . . . .' The story continued, Liz looking at me with growing disbelief. Finally she could not stand any more.

'What do you mean?' she yelled in indignation. 'Of course you're making mistakes — you're no saint!' I stopped moaning and looked resentfully at her, ready to argue in the opposite direction if pressed further. But she continued, forcing me to see something which had never occurred to me before. 'You seem to be noticing only the retrograde steps. But you're conveniently forgetting how very far you've gone. You've made tremendous progress — I can see it. If you're going back one step, you're also going forward the proverbial two, every time!'

She was right. It is always the simplest thing that we cannot see for ourselves. Someone else has to tell us. Life, apparently, is like that. All those years I had been noticing only the failures, jumping back into my box and waiting for the next, inevitable new start which would, of course, make everything all right and let me prove to myself that I was a successful human being. I had been ignoring all the achievements. I must have been at this point that I finally let the sun shine in.

Kate, also, was a very important factor in the search for self-acceptance. More than Sloopy had ever been, she has become a real person in my life, absolutely faithful, perpetually loving and a born clown. She taught me to laugh again, with all her antics; she doubles my enjoyment of everything that is happening -- because I share it all with her; she taught me to care.

She could clear a six-foot wall if she thought it worth her while. We used to play a game where I could hold a stick at arm's length and she would leap up to catch it. We did it once too often. She came down crookedly, I heard a crack like a pistol-shot and a single scream. Kate's leg was broken. The thigh part was splintered in three places as the X-ray showed. The first vet said nothing could be done — she must be put straight out of her pain. The next vet suggested amputation. Finally I found a vet who offered to operate. For two days I was extremely calm and sensible while she, my companion through such good and bad times, was having a plate and screws put on the critical fracture. But when it was all over and she was sleeping soundly in her basket, I experienced T L E almost continually for the next thirty-six hours. The bill cleared out my bank account, but Kate recovered.

Somehow I don't think there will ever be an end to all the amazing, horrifying, exciting, awful and ridiculous things that happen to me. I keep thinking that personal freedom, emancipation, joy and liberation from stigma must surely have reached their limit. But always there are new discoveries and further adjustments to be made. Do I get irritated with other people around for too long? Then I learn to live alone. This prevents the confusion and fatigue caused by too much head-on confrontation in what most people would call normal conversation. Do I have too many showdowns with too many bosses at work? Well — I learn to work alone. Am I always bumping my head? That is no problem — I have a pretty thick skull. So I'm always spilling my tea in my lap? (Often caused by shaking due to drug-poisoning when all those drugs reach a toxic level in my blood.) So I become a tea stain removal expert. Do I need someone to talk to? Well — I get a dog with a mind of her own. And does music precipitate T L E? Then it must be rationed.

If sleep and regular food are essential, then life must be arranged to accommodate that, also. Am I a loner? Then learn to enjoy it! I used to think that being a loner was unnatural, that I was still basically ashamed to be with people. But that is just not true. Many people prefer to be alone, beginning with Greta Garbo. The non-gregarious types simply have different personal requisites from other people. There is no problem or situation that an epileptic or anyone else for that matter, cannot solve themselves quite simply, with a little thought.

Life is good, now, and full of happenings. For example, on a recent escapade, I visited one of the many Devil's Punchbowls near Aberystwyth. There was nobody around at 7.30 a.m. so Kate and I nipped over the wall to have a cold bath in one of the devil's smaller wine glasses. Then we went exploring. I found a rusty, disused ladder leading down to the biggest pool under the falls. Kate, clever as she is, could not negotiate that ladder so she would have to be carried. I threw my travelling bag down first. It contained this manuscript. No prizes for the one who guesses where it landed — smack in the middle of that old devil's alcoholic beverage.

Round and round it went, sinking lower each time. Kate, now eighteen months old and faithful to the end, thought it was me and dived straight in, tail, head and feet spread wide, like a flying fox. Round and round she went, getting no nearer to the doomed bag and manuscript.

Over the waterfall went the bag, closely followed by a yelping, bedraggled, black and white sheepdog. Another twenty feet down. In between hysterics, I vowed that if the manuscript and bag were recovered readable, I would finish it — and all devils be damned. Bag and Kate were both hauled out fifty feet down.

Not a soul had seen us as the tourists had not started 'doing' Devil's Bridge that day. So I poured everything out of the bag and laid it on the rocks to dry — nightdress, cardigan, towel, face-washer, socks, swimsuit, sunhat, sunglasses, pills, (I was measuring out tegretol in granules for weeks) and the manuscript, not much the worse for its wash.

Bless Kate. Bless all who have got me even this far. This ragged owlet has taken itself off the hoarding and swung into the blue sky, performing like a new swallow. No more branding for me.

Epilogue

There is an uncertainty about life for an epileptic which could become irksome if not met head on. Tonight I may have a fit in my sleep. That means I'll awaken tomorrow with a bitten tongue, a wet pillow, a stiff neck and a brain that is working like a car on three cylinders which are firing out of order. I can handle that now. Or, perhaps tomorrow, while shopping, I'll have a *grand mal* in the line at Tesco's. Some of those around me will be frightened, some will be disgusted for the wrong reasons — and probably at least one person will understand and take over. I hope they don't call an ambulance. I hope I don't upset too many people. Whatever happens, I'll survive and the terrors of the black ocean which close over me will evaporate. Maybe, the next day, I will spend an entire afternoon in a state of T L E and nothing will get done properly. It will have to be done again, that's all. And possibly none of these things will happen. Maybe . . . maybe I will never have a *grand mal* again.

No epileptic need be helpless and most epileptics can have total independence — if they really want it. There is no reason why we should not marry and have children — a careful consultation with a specialist should confirm that. So let yourself fall in love . . . and take the consequences! There is no need to shield yourself from everything for fear of a few accidents.

There are bound to be accidents, but the joys of a full life more than make up for a little pain and fear. Don't let yourself get into a situation of over-protection. You are quite capable of picking yourself up. And above all, don't get convinced that you are special, different or set apart from the rest of mankind. If you are mean and nasty

188

and unlovable, nobody will love you; if you are generous and patient and kind, everybody will. It is the same for all human beings. So whatever it is you want to do, from growing cucumbers to swimming in the Olympics, dive in and do it — you can and you will. I know it.

Other Arrow Books of interest:

FOR THE LOVE OF ANN
James Copeland

'The doctor cleared his throat and spoke very quietly. "I am so sorry to have to tell you this, but I'm afraid that our tests show that it is extremely unlikely that your daughter will ever be educated, or for that matter, that she will ever be able to recognize you as her parents." '

That was in 1958 and Ann Hodges was six years and eight months old. Today that same girl is in her twenties, full of charm, devoted to her parents and her brothers and excitedly taking in the world and its challenges.

Between those two dates lies a remarkable story. A love story born out of hopelessness and ignorance and nurtured in years of tears and joy . . .

ALL FOR THE LOVE OF ANN

55p

HEDINGHAM HARVEST

Geoffrey Robinson

For years Geoffrey Robinson has recorded his family's accounts of village life in Lincolnshire. Based on these memories, *Hedingham Harvest* is a cheerful, affectionate and often hilarious chronicle of life and love in a Victorian village.

'A delightfully lively, graphic and captivating chronicle of village life' *Sunday Express*

'Marvellous . . . unique of its kind' *Guardian*

85p